SKIN CARE

THIS BOOK INCLUDES:
"BODY BUTTER RECIPES" AND "BODY SCRUBS"
INEXPENSIVE HOMEMADE RECIPES AND NATURAL REMEDIES FOR LIFTING AND REJUVENATED SKIN

AMANDA CARE

SKIN CARE

SKIN CARE:

This book includes:

"Body Butter Recipes" and "Body Scrubs":

Inexpensive, Homemade Recipes And Natural Remedies

For Luminous And Rejuvenated Skin!

Amanda Care

SKIN CARE

THIS BOOK INCLUDES

BOOK 1: 14 (PAGE)
BODY BUTTER RECIPES
SIMPLE DIY RECIPES TO MAKE SOFT AND GLOW YOUR SKIN WITH HOMEMADE BODY BUTTER

BOOK 2: 128 (PAGE)
BODY SCRUB RECIPES
EASY AND NATURAL DIY RECIPES TO MAKE HOMEMADE BODY SCRUBS FOR SMOOTH, SOFT AND YOUTHFUL SKIN

© Copyright 2020 by Amanda Care - All rights reserved.

The content contained within this book may not be reproduced, duplicated or transmitted without direct written permission from the author or the publisher.

Under no circumstances will any blame or legal responsibility be held against the publisher, or author, for any damages, reparation, or monetary loss due to the information contained within this book. Either directly or indirectly.

Legal Notice:

This book is copyright protected. This book is only for personal use. You cannot amend, distribute, sell, use, quote or paraphrase any part, or the content within this book, without the consent of the author or publisher.

Disclaimer Notice:

Please note the information contained within this document is for educational and entertainment purposes only. All effort has been executed to present accurate, up to date, and reliable, complete information. No warranties of any kind are declared or implied. Readers acknowledge that the author is not engaging in the rendering of legal, financial, medical or professional advice. The content within this book has been derived from various sources. Please consult a licensed professional before attempting any techniques outlined in this book.

By reading this document, the reader agrees that under no circumstances is the author responsible for any losses, direct or indirect, which are incurred as a result of the use of information contained within this document, including, but not limited to, — errors, omissions, or inaccuracies.

SKIN CARE

BODY BUTTER Recipes

SIMPLE DIY RECIPES TO MAKE SOFT AND GLOW YOUR SKIN WITH HOMEMADE BODY BUTTER

AMANDA CARE

SKIN CARE

BODY BUTTER RECIPES

Simple Diy Recipes To Make Soft And Glow Your Skin With Homemade Body Butter

Amanda Care

SKIN CARE

TABLE OF CONTENTS

INTRODUCTION..**14**

CHAPTER 1 WHAT ARE BODY BUTTERS?...**22**

CHAPTER 2 INGREDIENTS OF BODY BUTTER..**28**

CHAPTER 3 BODY BUTTER BASICS AND SOME BASIC RECIPES **36**

CHAPTER 4 MOISTURIZING BODY BUTTERS...**48**

CHAPTER 5 BASIC BODY BUTTER RECIPES **58**

CHAPTER 6 BODY BUTTER RECIPES FOR SPECIFIC PURPOSES **74**

CHAPTER 7 COMPLICATED BODY BUTTER RECIPES...................................**84**

CHAPTER 8 BODY BUTTER RECIPES FOR DIFFERENT KINDS OF SKIN....**94**

CHAPTER 9 MORE COMPLICATED BODY BUTTER RECIPES AND REGIMENS **104**

CHAPTER 10 WHAT YOU NEED TO LEARN ABOUT ORGANIC ESSENTIAL OILS............**116**

CONCLUSION..**118**

Introduction

We all want to look and feel our best, but at what price are we paying for our pursuit of beauty? There are hundreds of thousands of commercial body care products out there; from creams, lotions and body scrubs to make-up and deodorant, all available in your supermarket, online and even in natural food markets. Most of them claim to soften our skin, improve our appearance or make us smell great, but the majority of these products contain toxic chemicals, synthetic preservatives, artificial fragrances, colors and mineral oils which are all too often animal-tested before making it to the shelf.

Many of us use an average of over 10 body care products daily, bombarding our bodies with hundreds of different chemicals each day. Over 10,000 Ingredients: can be used to make these products, including harsh substances like formaldehyde, carcinogens, parabens, plus a cocktail of other synthetic Ingredients: and toxins. While many of these elements can be irritating to the skin itself, they can also be absorbed into our bloodstream causing sensitivities and potential long-term health risks. The skin is our largest organ, after all, so we need to be aware that what we apply on our skin can and will end up inside our bodies.

Ninety percent of personal care products contain Sodium Lauryl Sulfate (SLS). This is a known skin, lung and eye irritant that interacts and combines with other chemicals to form nitrosamines—which are mostly carcinogenic. Parabens, also found in personal care products such as deodorants, shampoos, make-up and lotions, contain estrogen-mimicking properties that have been linked to breast cancer (Byford, 2002; Pugazhendhi, 2007). And the list goes on.

You Can Stop the Toxic Cycle

Fortunately, there is a way to look radiant and beautiful while still having the peace of mind knowing that you are not damaging your skin and compromising your health each day. With a little help from nature, you can take your health into your own hands while consciously caring for your beautiful body, the animals and the environment. This plant-based body care system not only ensures that no animals were harmed in product testing or manufacturing, it also means that no toxic substances are going onto your skin and into your body. By merely using organic body care ingredients, you are taking a big step toward a healthier and more sustainable lifestyle.

I will empower you to treat yourself to a youthful, radiant glow from the inside out, using the nutritive and organic Ingredients: that your skin deserves. Featuring all-natural Ingredients: such as flowers, oil blends and fresh fruits, I have researched and formulated these replenishing recipes to prove to you that harmful, synthetic chemicals are not necessary to enjoy a glowing, healthy look and feel. You can create these recipes in your own home with simple Ingredients: and equipment from your kitchen, garden or pantry.

The Benefits of Homemade Organic Skin & Body Care

Firstly, I'd like to share something with you. For a long time, I was suffering from low energy levels, high allergen levels and felt as though my mind was in a constant fog. Not finding the answers to my many questions about why I was feeling this way through traditional means or prescribed antidotes, I began researching the effects of natural and organic Ingredients: on a person's physical and mental well-being. By simply cutting the amount of toxins I put in and on my body, I noticed an increase in my energy levels, my allergies were alleviated plus my mind (and my skin!) were evident.

Your Skin Will Thank You

The benefits of using homemade organic body care can be felt and seen upon immediate use. Once you start making and using your own all-natural creations, you'll never look back to using commercial alternatives. The healing properties of homemade organic body care far outweigh those of their commercial and synthetic counterparts. They are anti-inflammatory, stimulating and soothing to the skin. Plus, they are loaded with anti-aging properties including antioxidants and vitamins to help achieve a youthful glow.

Cocoa butter adds calming relief for eczema and psoriasis, whereas commercial creams and lotions can be loaded with irritants. Many toxins in store-bought items will clog your pores inhibiting healthy skin; in contrast, diluted tangerine juice, with its antibacterial and antifungal properties, is an excellent ingredient for healthy pores without the risk of side effects. Preservatives in commercial body care products are sometimes the most toxic components. So, why put parabens and coal tar dyes on your body when natural Vitamin E Oil, with its antioxidant properties, can act as a preservative in your butters and lotions?

Other lifestyle choices can have an impact on your skin's health in conjunction with these organic body care recipes. For instance, it has been shown that a diet rich in plant-based foods (a colorful rainbow of fruits and vegetables), ample exercise, plenty of water and a reduction in your exposure to environmental pollutants (such as smoking) can positively contribute to your radiant glow.

It's Easy, Sustainable and Cost-Effective

Making your own organic body care products is not only healthy but practical. It's an affordable way to enjoy a luxurious skin care system, designed just for you, without spending money on expensive brands. Plus, you will always know precisely what Ingredients: are in your body care products and from where they were sourced.

Many of the Ingredients: used in making your own body care products will already be in your pantry while others can be purchased, often in bulk, at natural food markets or online. Depending on product availability and your personal budget, opt for Ingredients: labeled 'organic' whenever possible. By choosing organic, fewer toxins will be applied to your skin, and you will be supporting sustainable cultivation while helping the environment by lessening the impact of the chemical manufacturing industry.

It's Time to Experience a Healthy Glow

So when you walk down the aisle in the supermarket and look at the hundreds of body care products with additives like Sodium Lauryl Sulfate and Isopropyl Alcohol, you will be armed with the comfort and knowledge of having your own nutritive, gentle, all-natural products, that you created yourself, at home.

 Are you ready to ditch those chemicals and embrace your inner eco-chic beauty? I am sure you will love the benefits of these easy-to-follow organic body care recipes that will nourish your skin and invigorate your senses.

After trying and testing the various formulas, it's my aim to help you detoxify your body using effective, proven remedies and my hope is that you will find your own favorites among the recipes and tips—to enjoy for a lifetime. A healthy glow has never felt so beautiful.

Before You Begin

These recipes are formulated to be kind and gentle to your skin, but if you have any sensitivities or are concerned about any ingredients, a patch test is a quick and easy way to find out if your skin will react to a particular substance.

Try a Patch Test

Simply apply a small amount of the ingredient in question onto the center of a Band-Aid (see dilution guide for essential oils below). Then place it on the inside of your forearm. Leave it there for 24 hours. If the area becomes irritated before that time is up, take the Band-Aid off and rinse gently with cold water making sure not to scrub, as that may cause further discomfort. If the reaction does not subside seek help from a healthcare practitioner. After 24 hours, remove the Band-Aid and look for signs of redness, swelling or other irritation. If the skin looks healthy, the ingredient should be safe to use. If you find yourself sensitive, you can personalize the recipe by replacing the ingredient with another natural alternative.

Using Essential Oils

Essential oils are highly concentrated and extracted from the leaves and roots of various plants, with various therapeutic, aromatic and cosmetic uses. Due to their high potency and concentration, it is essential to use them correctly and sparingly. Avoid the use of undiluted or highly concentrated essential oils directly on the skin unless indicated; lavender is one of the few essential oils that can be used 'neat', or directly on the skin undiluted, a drop or two at a time. If performing a patch test, ensure to dilute as per the chosen recipe. As a general rule, 1 drop of essential oil should be diluted with 5ml of carrier oil before being applied to the skin. Do not ingest essential oils and keep out of reach of children and pets. Ensure essential oils do not come into contact with your eyes and use with caution if you are pregnant, planning to become pregnant or have any pre-existing medical conditions.

Diluting with Carrier Oils

Carrier oils are vegetable-derived oils that can be used in your body care recipes as a base or to dilute essential oils before being applied on the skin. These oils can be alternated, combined, or used in place of one another depending on availability, therapeutic or textural preference, or skin sensitivities. Some people may find themselves sensitive to coconut oil, for example, so replacing it with sweet almond oil may work as an adequate substitute. Experimenting with various carrier oils can help establish what works best for you. Some popular carrier oil varieties include:

- For a light to medium consistency: Sweet almond oil, apricot kernel oil, grapeseed oil, jojoba oil, sunflower oil, argan oil
- For a medium to dense consistency: Avocado oil, coconut oil (virgin), olive oil, hazelnut oil, macadamia oil, rosehip oil, sesame oil

Alternatively, you can also use thicker plant-based butters, such as cocoa butter (fluffy consistency) or shea butter (a slightly sticky and solid mass before warming or mixing with other Ingredients:) depending on the texture you desire.

Be sure to store carrier oils and butters in a cool, dark place to extend their shelf life. Carrier oils should have a light, nutty aroma—if the oil has a strong, bitter aroma it may have gone rancid.

Keeping your Pores Clog-Free

Many oils contain attractive benefits for our skin, but when using oil (or any ingredient) on our skin you have to consider whether it is comedogenic, meaning, likely to clog pores. If you are prone to comedogenic reactions (i.e. bumpiness on the skin, acne or irritation after applying certain oils), it's essential to familiarize yourself with various Ingredients: to understand the relationship your skin has with it.

Some heavier oils such as olive oil, for example, may clog pores for those with sensitive or acne-prone skin and are better used as a wash or scrub to minimize clogging effects. Whereas jojoba oil and argan oil tend to work well with most skin-types and can even alleviate acne. These reactions can vary from person to person—what may work fine for some people might pose as an issue for others. There are no definite results so you will need to make a personalized decision and evaluate which oils work best with your skin type. Whichever oils you choose, always look for organic and 100% pure with no added nasties.

Keep in mind that some of the Ingredients: in these recipes are interchangeable. You can make alterations to accommodate to your skin type, to suit your personal preferences or to utilize what you have on hand.

Chapter 1 What are Body Butters?

What Are Body Butters?

You may not be aware of body butters. These are actually moisturizers that contain lubricating ingredients. They are technically like lotions, only better. These ingredients serve as a protective barrier or a shield so that moisture would stay within the skin and outside environmental elements that may be harmful to the skin would not be able to come in.

Body butters are more emollient, have high viscosity and more useful for those with dry skin. Some examples of these lubricating Ingredients: are shea butter, coconut oil, olive and jojoba oils. Consumers also describe body butters as ensuring a "more luxurious" feel on their skin.

Body butters are extra moisturizing because they contain less water and have more essential oils or butters needed by the body to maintain moisture. Viscosity and consistency are higher so these butters are placed in jars where they would be scooped, because it would be difficult to pump them out.

Another wonder of body butter is it is ideal for those with sensitive skin. Allergies or rashes seldom occur because the Ingredients: of body butters are all-natural. Usually, a body butter is made up of an oil base and a few more Ingredients:. You would appreciate the fact that they are free from various chemicals and preservatives that could harm your skin.

Body Lotion Vs. Body Butter

Body lotion and body butter are the two most commonly used skin moisturizers. While both of them are effective in keeping your skin radiant and soft, these two products have their own unique qualities and features. In order to protect your skin better, you need to know the difference between the two moisturizers.

Lotions

Products that are identified as lotions have a lighter consistency compared to body butters. They also have meager oil percentage, and they cannot lubricate the skin. This one can accommodate every type of skin available. Lotions are also considered as humectants because they are effective at preserving the existing moisture in the body. These products usually contain alpha hydroxyl as well as hyaluronic acid. These are powerful substances that can remove dead cells from the upper layers of the skin, draw out the natural waters found in the dermis, and then send it to the epidermis.

Body lotions are highly recommended products for the hot summer months because these can keep you moisturized without making your skin too sticky and greasy. However, their light consistency does not make them ideal products for people who have dry skin.

Body Butters

Moisturizers that are considered as butters tend to be a little bit denser and highly emollient. These products are occlusive, which means that they create a protective coating on the skin. This particular coat is like a barrier that defends your skin against external aggressors such as dust particles and harmful UV rays. In addition, it also helps retain moisture in your body for an extended period of time. Body butter is highly recommended for people who have dehydrated skin because these are thicker and more viscous than creams and lotions.

Aside from acting as a moisturizer, body butter also helps rejuvenate your skin, reduce the wrinkles or visible lines on your face, and make you look extremely younger. This is an ideal product during the cold winter months because it keeps your skin moisturized for an extended period of time.

If you have oily skin, it is not recommended that you use body butter all the time. The protective barrier that it creates tends to block out your pores, thus making your skin an excellent breeding ground for bacteria.

Different Uses of Body Butter

Aside from being a moisturizing agent, body butter can actually be used in several different ways. Check these out below:

Hand Care – you can use body butter to keep your hands soft. You just need to apply small amounts of this product every day so that your fingers will stay moisturized all the time. If your hands are quite dry, apply large quantities of it before you go to bed. For better results, you can also put on a pair of cotton gloves while you sleep.

Smoothing out Dry Patches – if you have flaky elbows or toes, then this product is perfect for you. All you have to do is apply small quantities of body butter on the dry regions of your skin. Afterwards, massage it a little bit so that it can easily be absorbed by the body.

Foot Care – After thoroughly washing your feet, massage them with body butter on a daily basis to them supple and soft. It is also recommended that you apply large amounts of this product on your feet, cover them with cotton socks overnight. This simple treatment can rejuvenate your skin quickly.

Cuticle Softener – slather some of this butter on your fingers and toes to make it easier for you to remove your cuticles.

Eye Makeup Remover – roll a dampened cotton ball on a piece of body butter. Then, lightly scrub off the makeup. This can also be used to remove water-proof mascara, as well as maintaining the beauty of your eyelashes.

Face moisturizer – Work a small amount of body butter on your hands before applying it. Afterwards, lightly massage your face using upward strokes. Stroke your palms across your forehead. Then, slightly pinch your jaw line. Finally, apply using upward strokes on your cheeks. Regularly massaging your face will surely remove your wrinkles and fine lines.

Décolletage Moisturizer – smear some of the butter on your neck. Use upward strokes to massage your neck. Repeat this process on a daily basis.

Aftershave and leg balm – body butter also removes the "fish scales" that you acquire after shaving.

Lip Balm – Apply this product similar to how you do it with other types of lip balm.

Massage – Had an incredibly stressful day? Body butter offers a soothing and relaxing feeling to your body too.

Do you want to know another wonder of body butter? You could actually make your own body butters right in the comfort of your home. They are easy to make, and the Ingredients: are not that hard to find.

Are you ready for a healthier skin? Find out more about making your own body butters.

SKIN CARE

Chapter 2 Ingredients of Body Butter

There are many different Ingredients: that go into natural beauty products, so it is essential to know the properties of the Ingredients: you will be using and why they are necessary. We will briefly cover essential oils and moisturizing ingredients, such as emollients and humectants; as well as the less natural but more functional Ingredients: such as emulsifiers, detergents/surfactants, preservatives, and antioxidants.

Essential oils

Essential oils are not really "oils" as such, but highly volatile compounds extracted from fruits, flowers, leaves, roots, woods, and resins, mainly by steam distillation (or expression, in the case of citrus oils). Those materials too delicate to be distilled are usually made into an absolute by either solvent extraction (such as rose absolute and jasmine absolute) or C02 extraction. As they are quite volatile and adversely affected by heat, essential oils should always be added at the cooling stage of any recipes that involve heating.

Extremely concentrated essential oils should never be used undiluted on the skin, as they can cause minor to quite significant irritation. There are many oils that are contraindicated during pregnancy due to their emmenagogue (brings on menstruation) action, though as a general rule I would avoid all essential oils during the first trimester and consult an aromatherapist specializing in pregnancy and birth during later months when aromatherapy can be beneficial.

Dosages

Dosages of essential oils in different product types can vary, but I generally follow the following rules:

- Facial skincare products—a few drops per 3½fl oz (100ml) of the product up to a maximum of 0.5%. I have pretty sensitive skin on my face, so I tend to avoid using more than a couple of drops in a facial moisturizer.

- Rinse-off products, such as shower gels or soaps: 1–2%.

- Leave-on products, such as creams and lotions for the body: 1–2% depending on the oils used and the part of the body. Stick to 1% at first until you know how you will react to a particular oil.

Blending essential oils

When blending a fragrance for a product with essential oils, I consider two aspects: What therapeutic benefits, if any, do I want, and what kind of fragrance am I looking for?

There is absolutely no point in throwing together a bunch of oils that smell terrible when combined just because they are all good for a particular purpose. When I teach natural perfumery, I categorize the oils by both their fragrance family, such as citrus, woody, and floral, and by their volatility, or rate of evaporation—top, middle, and base notes. You will often find that fragrances that fall into the same categories have similar evaporation rates: for example, citrus oils all tend to be top notes, and all resins tend to be base notes. To get a balanced fragrance, it is a good idea to include oil from each of the top, middle, and base note ranges.

I have given suggested essential oil blends for all of the recipes, but do not feel you have to follow them. The fragrance is a very personal thing, so feel free to experiment. You do not need to buy lots of different essential oils since you can still make great fragrances with just a select few.

Herbal Ingredients:

It's incredibly quick to incorporate herbs to the homemade products. There are several types of herbal extracts that you can buy ready-made and some you can easily make yourself. Most commercial skincare products would use a standardized extract rather than adding fresh herbs in the form of an infusion since infusions do have a tendency to make some products unstable and go off more quickly. If you are making products just for yourself, this shouldn't be a problem, but make sure you do add a preservative when adding herbs to a water-based recipe.

Infusions

Creating an extract (or infusion) dependent on water from the leaves or blooming dried or fresh grass tops are as easy as creating a cup of herbal tea. Simply apply a heaped dried or minced tablespoon of fresh herbs to a cup or jug and dump on boiling water until it reaches the top. Cover with a saucer and require infusing with a tea strainer or a piece of fine cheesecloth (muslin) for 10 minutes before straining off the herb matter.

Dispose of the herbs, then apply the cooled liquid to your recipe at the appropriate point.

If you are making infusions in more significant quantities, add one teaspoon of herbs for each cup of water. Hold unpreserved herbal infusions in the refrigerator no more than a day, as they go off very quickly.

Flower waters

Another way to incorporate plant compounds from water into the items is by utilizing flower waters, or hydrolats. They are the by-products of natural oils steam distillation, which are very simple to use. The most common ones are lavender, orange flower, and rosewater. These also make great skin fresheners and maintain the properties of the essential oils from which they are produced.

Infused oils

When you produce an oil-based product, like a balm or salve, you will be able to macerate the herbs in the base oil used in the recipe. One of the best methods to get this accomplished is to place a heaped herbal teaspoon in a bowl and cover them with your preference of base oil. Put this over a hot water saucepan and cook for an hour, making sure the saucepan does not boil cold. Don't let the oil get overheated: the water should be simmering, rather than the oil. Strain the plant content and waste it, then retain the fat for your recipes. Alternatively buy ready-made infused oils from a retailer of herbs.

Tinctures, glycerols & C02 extracts

These final kinds of extracts are too hard for most of us to make at home and are better obtained from a reputable manufacturer of herbs.

Tinctures are produced by macerating herbs in a Tinctures for a relatively long period of time, created by macerating herbs in a combination of alcohol and water for a relatively long time. They are sold primarily for internal use by herbalists, but they are added to their products by many skin care companies. Tinctures may be inappropriate for use in sensitive skin goods because of their alcohol content, as they can have quite a drying effect. Instead, the way around this is using glycerol (glycerin extract). A glycerol's benefit is that the herb is macerated into both water-soluble and humectant glycerin. This ensures it is ideal for water-based products as well as those with an emulsifier, such as creams and lotions. Stick to using oil macerates in products containing only oils and waxes (or an emulsifier) since glycerin is not soluble in oil alone. CO2 extracts are the product of a relatively new (and costly) method, known as supercritical CO2 extraction, used to produce herbal and plant extracts for use in the cosmetics, food and herbal industries. Under high pressure, the plant material is flooded with carbon dioxide, which serves as a solution for removing the plant's fragile materials. Because of the lower temperatures required, this is used as a way to extract essential plant oils, without chemical solvents when distillation of steam is difficult. It is also used for producing extracts of herbs which can be applied to your items. Vanilla C02 extract is especially useful since pure vanilla is not soluble in oil and is hard to integrate into goods, while the C02 extract works perfectly.

MOISTURIZING INGREDIENTS:

There are three forms of moisturizing Ingredients: that are used in creams or lotions — emollients, occlusive, and humectants— and the task is to mix them to best effect. Understanding their essential functions and how they operate together will make making your own recipes from scratch, or changing any of the recipes, much more manageable.

Emollients

Such help in enhancing the texture of the skin by softening, smoothing, and growing its versatility. These will be pure vegetable oils and butter for my recipes, varying from very light and easily absorbed oils like a thistle to thicker, healthier butter like coconut and shea. Many oils, such as borage and hemp, are high in essential fatty acids and vitamins but are not extraordinarily emollient. On their own, they can feel freezing. That's why it's essential to include a few different oils in each recipe, to improve the performance and skin feel. I have included detail on the oils for each product, so you'll get a good idea of what works on different types of skin.

Occlusive

These minimize trans-epidermal water loss (TEWL) by forming a waterproof layer over the skin. When added to slightly damp skin, they work better. Many emollients, such as cocoa butter, have occlusive properties, along with waxes such as beeswax, making them ideal for creating protective materials that shield the skin from the elements. Many occlusives are quite comedogenic (aggravating acne) and should be prevented on spot-or acne-prone skin types.

Most skincare experts dislike occlusive additives, as it is thought that they hinder the skin from breathing; nevertheless, they are ideal for certain places, such as eyes, hands and feet, to build a protective barrier on dry, cracked skin.

Humectants

humectants are made of glycerine, sugar, and hyaluronic acid. While humectants are indeed moisturizers, they function in a different way than other moisturizers by drawing water to the skin to hold cells hydrated and plump. Once the water is drawn to the surface, extra additives, such as emollients and occlusives, are required to keep it in place.

EMULSIFIERS & DETERGENTS

Products such as body butter, lip balms, and balms are fairly easy to manufacture for the treatment, and suitable goods may usually be manufactured to make them 100 per cent sustainable today. However, if you want to produce a more complex cream or lotion, you will need to use both an emulsifier to blend the oil and water-based products, and a preservative to protect them from falling off.

Emulsifiers

In simplistic terms, the function of an emulsifier is to make the oil-soluble Ingredients: deal with water-soluble Ingredients:; likewise, that when making mayonnaise, you can apply egg yolk to the oil and vinegar. It happens because there is lecithin in egg yolk which has emulsifying powers. If you're creating a lotion or cream, you'd also need to use a thickener to get the feel perfect, as just an emulsifier will make a milky substance alone. Many natural emulsifiers you might purchase have thickening properties, but you'd need to add an extra component in most situations.

Emulsifying wax

The most widely used and easy-to-use emulsifier for home use is emulsifying wax, which for a variety of different formulae is a popular term. Some emulsifying wax styles include thickeners, and some don't — if you're not sure to ask your manufacturer, or just follow a formula. If it is too small and watery, a different thickener can need to be used.

Using emulsifying wax

I find that using emulsifying wax at 25 per cent of the total fat content without butter or thickeners produces a lotion that is dense, but still pourable. When you choose to make a thicker mixture, then add a little more emulsifying wax to the formula or introduce some cetyl alcohol.

The alternatives to emulsifying wax

Besides emulsifying wax, many emulsifiers are accessible to the home crafter in the food industry, and you may choose to use these instead — or at least play with them. I noticed that replacing 5 per cent emulsifying wax with 5 per cent glyceryl monostearate plus 2–3 per cent cetyl alcohol works fine for most of the recipes.

Chapter 3 Body Butter Basics and Some Basic Recipes

Body butter is intended to be as decadent as it sounds. It provides your skin with a full blast of moisture, thanks to the high oil content. Body butters differ from lotions in that they are much thicker and can provide your skin with a thicker barrier against moisture loss.

Body butters have been known since Roman times. Those body butters are similar in composition to the recipes provided in that the Ingredients: are all natural without the harmful preservatives found in commercial products. We've used a variety of butters including shea butter, mango butter, and coconut butter as the base for our body butter recipes. These butters contain essential vitamins and antioxidants that are not only replenishing, but also healing. The high viscosity levels make the butters quite dense and perfect for very dry areas. It is also a good idea to give your whole body the body butter treatment once a week to get amazingly soft, supple skin all over.

Benefits Of Body Butter

Body butters provide ultimate moisturizing for ultimate beauty. They are composed of humectants and occlusive agents like body lotions. Still, the composition in butters comes in at a ratio that takes their effect on the skin right off the charts.

Common humectants found in body butter include honey and glycerine. These do the heavy lifting when it comes to luring moisture from the air into your skin.

Common occlusives include shea butter and silicone. The occlusives are your official skin guards, which ensure that once the moisture has made its way into your skin, it stays there.

Storage

Use mason jars or another type of jar with an airtight lid to store your body butters. You should sterilize the jars in a water bath before filling and sealing them. Once sealed, store them in a cool place.

How To Do It Yourself

Body butters are simple to make at home and require little time. Standard body butters include a combination of the following elements:

Butter

Oil

Essential oil

What To Watch Out For

The thick consistency of body butter means you need to use jars for storage, and of course, that means contamination is possible. It is best to store your butter in smaller jars so the chance of contamination per jar is less. Also ensure that you have clean, dry hands before you stick your hand into one of the jars to scoop out some body butter or use a clean spoon.

Body Butter Recipes

1. Hawaiian Body Butter

Slather summer on your body with this body butter scented with pineapple and mango. The mango butter is wonderfully rich. Its anti-aging properties can reduce those irritating lines that begin to appear as you age. The mango butter combined with coconut oil and Vitamin E will have you feeling lovely and soft.

Makes: 12 ounces

Ingredients:

1 teaspoon pineapple essential oil

½ cup mango butter

1 cup coconut oil

1 teaspoon vitamin E oil

Directions:

Place the Ingredients: in a glass bowl and beat until smooth.

Scoop the butter into sterilized jars and store it in a cool place.

Mandarin Chocolate Body Butter

Raise your hands if you love the heavenly scent of mandarin spiked with chocolate! This body butter is fantastic on the skin. The natural scents provide a mood boost that will have you whipping through the morning and afternoon in a sweet haze.

Makes: 12 ounces

Ingredients: 1 teaspoon mandarin zest   1 teaspoon cocoa essential oil

1 ½ cups coconut butter*

Directions:

Place the Ingredients: in a glass bowl and beat them until smooth.

Scoop the butter into sterilized jars and store it in a cool place.

*Note: You can make your coconut butter by processing unsweetened, shredded coconut in a food processor until it is completely smooth.

Strawberry Vanilla Butter

Stay sweet all day long with lovely strawberry-and-vanilla-infused butter. Strawberries contain ellagic acid, which helps spur the production of collagen and in turn ensures you age more slowly. As in the case of raspberry seed essential oil, there is no such thing as strawberry essential oil, so you must be sure to purchase only strawberry seed essential oil to ensure you're getting an all-natural product.

Makes: 16 ounces

Ingredients: 2 teaspoons strawberry seed essential oil 1 cup shea butter ½ cup coconut oil ½ cup jojoba oil

Directions:

Fill a saucepan halfway up with water and heat over medium.

Grab a glass bowl that will fit over the mouth of the saucepan.

Place the shea butter and coconut oil in the glass bowl and stir until they are melted. Remove the bowl and place it on a cool surface. Add the oils, stir, and cool the mixture in the refrigerator for half an hour.

Once the mixture is cool, use a hand immersion blender to beat the butter until it is creamy.

Scoop the butter into clean jars with airtight lids and store it in a cool place until use.

Golden Body Butter

Oh, how she glows, and she glows. You will glow after using this butter, thanks to the cocoa powder and honey combination, which creates a slightly sun-kissed look.

Makes: 16 ounces

Ingredients:

2 tablespoons cocoa powder

2 tablespoons raw honey

1 cup shea butter

½ cup coconut oil

½ cup jojoba oil

Directions:

Fill a saucepan halfway up with water and heat it over medium.

Grab a glass bowl that will fit over the mouth of the saucepan.

Place the shea butter and coconut oil in the glass bowl and stir until melted.

Remove the bowl and place it on a cool surface.

Add the remaining ingredients, stir, and cool the mixture in the refrigerator for half an hour. Once it is cool, use a hand immersion blender to beat the butter until it is creamy.

Scoop the butter into clean jars with airtight lids and store them in a cool place until use.

Mango Body Butter

This simple, rich butter is great to use in the winter. After taking a shower, slather it all over your feet, don your socks, and wake up in the morning with feet so soft you'll feel as though you can float!

Makes: 14 ounces

Ingredients:

1 cup mango butter

½ cup coconut oil

1 teaspoon vitamin E oil

2 tablespoons aloe gel

Directions:

Fill a saucepan halfway up with water and heat it over medium.

Grab a glass bowl that will fit over the mouth of the saucepan.

Place the mango butter and coconut oil in the glass bowl and stir until it melts.

Remove the bowl and place it on a cool surface.

Add the remaining ingredients, stir, and cool the mixture in the refrigerator for half an hour. Once the mixture is cool, use a hand immersion blender to beat the butter until it is creamy.

Scoop the butter into clean jars with airtight lids and store it in a cool place until use.

Cinnamon Body Butter

The comfy scent of cinnamon can make you feel at home wherever you are. When used in a lotion, it will give you that same feeling of cozy comfort. With its anti-bacterial properties, cinnamon is also wonderful for the skin. It's soothing for the joints as well as the skin.

Makes: 12 ounces

Ingredients:

1 cup cocoa butter

½ cup argan oil

1 teaspoon cinnamon essential oil

1 teaspoon Arabica seed oil

Directions:

Fill a saucepan halfway up with water and heat it over medium.

Grab a glass bowl that will fit over the mouth of the saucepan.

Place the cocoa butter and coconut oil in the glass bowl and stir until they are melted.

Remove the bowl and place it on a cool surface.

Add the remaining ingredients, stir, and cool in refrigerator for half an hour.

Once the mixture is cool, use a hand immersion blender to beat the butter until it is creamy.

Scoop the butter into jars with airtight lids and store in a cool place until use.

Citrus Body Butter For Glowing Skin

Tea tree oil is an anti-bacterial, and the extra virgin coconut oil and shea butter will provide your skin with the moisture it needs throughout the day. The orange essential oil will keep your mind fresh and alert.

Makes: 35 ounces.

Ingredients:

3 cups extra virgin coconut oil

10 ½ ounces shea butter

5 drops tea tree oil

20 drops sweet orange essential oil

20 drops lemon essential oil

Directions:

Mix the shea butter and coconut oil in a jar, such as a Mason jar. Cover the jar tightly with a lid.

Create a water bath in a saucepan and place the jar in the water. Allow all the Ingredients: to melt.

Remove the pot from the heat and add the tea tree oil and essential oils. Mix well and cool for about 30 minutes.

Freeze the mixture for 10-15 minutes or more. When the oils start solidifying, remove it from the freezer and whip it with a whisk until you get a light buttery consistency.

Spoon the butter into a clean jar. Close the lid tightly and place it in a cool, dry area.

Vanilla Bean Body Butter

This body butter will make you feel rejuvenated throughout the day, thanks to the pleasant and soothing aroma of vanilla. It also helps relax the body and mind. The cocoa butter helps to nourish the skin deeply, and the almond oil provides it with much-needed vitamin E.

Makes: 16 ounces

Ingredients:

1 cup raw cocoa butter

½ cup sweet almond oil

½ cup coconut oil

2 vanilla bean pods

Directions:

Combine the cocoa butter and coconut oil in a pan. Place the pan over low heat. When the ingredients are melted, remove it from the heat and set it aside to cool.

Grind the vanilla beans in a coffee grinder or food processor.

Add the sweet almond oil and ground vanilla beans to the cooled cocoa butter and coconut oil mixture. Mix well and freeze for about 20-25 minutes.

Whip the mixture in a food processor until buttery and creamy.

Scoop the butter into a glass jar with a lid. Refrigerate and use when necessary.

Aloe Vera Body Butter

Aloe vera soothes the skin and prevents skin inflammation. The three butters in this recipe will provide your skin with much-needed moisture and will keep it soft and supple. The essential oils will relax your mind and body. The grapeseed oil and beeswax will help prevent skin conditions like rashes, eczema, and acne.

Makes: 30 ounces

Ingredients:

6 ounces shea butter

4 ounces mango butter

2 ounces coconut butter

2 ounces coconut oil

6 ounces grapeseed oil

1-ounce beeswax

4 ounces distilled water

4 ounces aloe Vera gel

40 drops sweet orange essential oil

40 drops patchouli essential oil

20 drops lavender essential oil

Directions:

Sterilize your jars.

Mix the shea butter, mango butter, coconut butter, coconut oil, grapeseed oil, and beeswax in a heatproof glass bowl.

Create a water bath in a saucepan and place the bowl over the saucepan. Allow all the Ingredients: to melt.

Remove the mixture from the heat and let it cool for a while.

Place an immersion blender or hand mixer in the bowl. Let it run on low speed.

Slowly pour in the water and aloe vera gel. The mixture will become homogenous and creamy once you start blending. Continue blending until it mixes well.

Add the essential oils. Mix well until you reach the desired consistency.

Spoon the butter into the sterilized jars. Close the lids tightly and store in a cool and dry place.

SKIN CARE

Chapter 4 Moisturizing Body Butters

Guidelines for Moisturizing Your Skin

Before you start making the body butters, here are some key reminders when moisturizing your skin:

Always use mild soaps instead of harsh soaps. Harsh soaps usually do nothing for the skin but dry them out.

Take a good amount of healthy omega 3 fatty acids from animal sources such as fish or krill oil. They are better than the ones found in plants.

Don't wash your hands too frequently as you'll end up drying them out. Washing extract, the natural oils from your skin. Do this too frequently and you'll end up giving yourself more problems as you'll start to develop some cracks on your skin. This makes it easy for you to get bacterial infections.

Orange Almond And Mango Body Butter

Ingredients:

1 1/3 cup mango butter

2/3 cup almond oil

7 drops sweet orange essential oil

Directions:

In a double boiler melt the essential the butter and wax (if any).

Let it cool down to room temperature.

Add the liquid oils, essential oils and the rest of the Ingredients: and stir.

Using a mixer blend at low speed for the first minute and mix well.

Slowly move to high speed until you reach the volume and consistency that you want.

Store in a cool and dry place.

Jasmine And Olive Body Butter

Ingredients:

1 1/3 cup shea butter

2/3 cup olive oil

5 drops Jasmine essential oil

Directions:

In a double boiler melt the essential the butter and wax (if any).

Let it cool down to room temperature.

Add the liquid oils, essential oils and the rest of the Ingredients: and stir.

Using a mixer blend at low speed for the first minute and mix well.

Slowly move to high speed until you reach the volume and consistency that you want.

Store in a cool and dry place.

Cedar Wood And Coconut Body Butter

Ingredients:

1 ½ cup shea butter

1/2 cup coconut oil

5 drops cedar wood essential oil

Directions:

In a double boiler melt the essential the butter and wax (if any).

Let it cool down to room temperature.

Add the liquid oils, essential oils and the rest of the Ingredients: and stir.

Using a mixer blend at low speed for the first minute and mix well.

Slowly move to high speed until you reach the volume and consistency that you want.

Store in a cool and dry place.

Tangerine And Olive Oil Body Butter

Ingredients:

1 1/3 cup mango butter

2/3 cup olive oil - 8 drops tangerine essential oil

Directions:

In a double boiler melt the essential the butter and wax (if any).

Let it cool down to room temperature.

Add the liquid oils, essential oils and the rest of the Ingredients: and stir.

Using a mixer blend at low speed for the first minute and mix well.

Slowly move to high speed until you reach the volume and consistency that you want.

Store in a cool and dry place.

Roman Chamomile And Olive Oil Body Butter

Ingredients:

1 1/3 cup cocoa butter

2/3 cup extra-virgin coconut oil

10 drops Roman chamomile essential oil

Directions:

In a double boiler melt the essential the butter and wax (if any).

Let it cool down to room temperature.

Add the liquid oils, essential oils and the rest of the Ingredients: and stir.

Using a mixer blend at low speed for the first minute and mix well.

Slowly move to high speed until you reach the volume and consistency that you want.

Store in a cool and dry place.

Clary Sage And Coconut Body Butter

Ingredients:

1 1/3 cup shea butter

2/3 cup coconut oil

5-10 drops Clary Sage essential oil

Directions:

In a double boiler melt the essential the butter and wax (if any).

Let it cool down to room temperature.

Add the liquid oils, essential oils and the rest of the Ingredients: and stir.

Using a mixer blend at low speed for the first minute and mix well.

Slowly move to high speed until you reach the volume and consistency that you want.

Store in a cool and dry place.

Mandarin And Olive Oil Body Butter

Ingredients: 1 1/3 cup solid body butter 2/3 cup olive oil

5-10 drops Mandarin essential oil

Directions:

In a double boiler melt the essential the butter and wax (if any).

Let it cool down to room temperature.

Add the liquid oils, essential oils and the rest of the Ingredients: and stir.

Using a mixer blend at low speed for the first minute and mix well.

Slowly move to high speed until you reach the volume and consistency that you want.

Store in a cool and dry place.

Rosemary Coconut And Olive Oil Body Butter

Ingredients:

1 1/3 cup mango butter

1/3 cup olive oil

1/3 cup extra virgin coconut oil

5-10 drops rosemary essential oil

Directions:

In a double boiler melt the essential the butter and wax (if any).

Let it cool down to room temperature.

Add the liquid oils, essential oils and the rest of the Ingredients: and stir.

Using a mixer blend at low speed for the first minute and mix well.

Slowly move to high speed until you reach the volume and consistency that you want.

Store in a cool and dry place.

Neroli Olive And Macadamia Nut Body Butter

Ingredients:

1 1/3 cup shea butter   1/3 cup macadamia nut oil   1/3 cup olive oil

5-10 drops Neroli essential oil

Directions:

In a double boiler melt the essential the butter and wax (if any).

Let it cool down to room temperature.

Add the liquid oils, essential oils and the rest of the Ingredients: and stir.

Using a mixer blend at low speed for the first minute and mix well.

Slowly move to high speed until you reach the volume and consistency that you want.

Store in a cool and dry place.

Vetiver And Peanut Oil Body Butter

Ingredients:

1 1/3 cup shea butter

2/3 cup peanut oil

5-10 drops Vetiver essential oil

Directions:

In a double boiler melt the essential the butter and wax (if any).

Let it cool down to room temperature.

Add the liquid oils, essential oils and the rest of the Ingredients: and stir.

Using a mixer blend at low speed for the first minute and mix well.

Slowly move to high speed until you reach the volume and consistency that you want.

Store in a cool and dry place.

Lemon Olive And Macadamia Nut Oil Body Butter

Ingredients:

1 1/3 cup cocoa butter 1/3 cup macadamia nut oil 1/3 cup olive oil

5-10 drops lemon essential oil

Directions:

In a double boiler melt the essential the butter and wax (if any).

Let it cool down to room temperature.

Add the liquid oils, essential oils and the rest of the Ingredients: and stir.

Using a mixer blend at low speed for the first minute and mix well.

Slowly move to high speed until you reach the volume and consistency that you want.

Store in a cool and dry place.

Lavender And Coconut Oil Body Butter

Ingredients:

1 cup cocoa butter 1/3 cup beeswax

2/3 cup extra virgin coconut oil

5-10 drops lavender essential oil

Directions:

In a double boiler melt the essential the butter and wax (if any).

Let it cool down to room temperature.

Add the liquid oils, essential oils and the rest of the Ingredients: and stir.

Using a mixer blend at low speed for the first minute and mix well.

Slowly move to high speed until you reach the volume and consistency that you want.

Store in a cool and dry place.

Rose And Jojoba Body Butter

Ingredients:

1 1/3 cup cocoa butter 2/3 cup jojoba oil

5-10 drops rose essential oil

Directions:

In a double boiler melt the essential the butter and wax (if any).

Let it cool down to room temperature.

Add the liquid oils, essential oils and the rest of the Ingredients: and stir.

Using a mixer blend at low speed for the first minute and mix well.

Slowly move to high speed until you reach the volume and consistency that you want.

Store in a cool and dry place.

Sandalwood And Olive Body Butter

Ingredients:

1 1/3 cup cocoa butter

2/3 cup extra virgin olive oil

5-10 drops Sandalwood essential oil

Directions:

In a double boiler melt the essential the butter and wax (if any).

Let it cool down to room temperature.

Add the liquid oils, essential oils and the rest of the Ingredients: and stir.

Using a mixer blend at low speed for the first minute and mix well.

Slowly move to high speed until you reach the volume and consistency that you want.

Store in a cool and dry place.

Jasmine And Rose Body Butter

Ingredients:

1 1/3 cup shea butter 2/3 cup olive oil 10 drops Jasmine essential oil

5 drops Rose essential oil

Directions:

In a double boiler melt the essential the butter and wax (if any).

Let it cool down to room temperature.

Add the liquid oils, essential oils and the rest of the Ingredients: and stir.

Using a mixer blend at low speed for the first minute and mix well.

Slowly move to high speed until you reach the volume and consistency that you want.

Store in a cool and dry place.

Juniper Berry Olive Body Butter

Ingredients:

1 1/3 cup cocoa butter ¼ cup grape seed oil

½ cup olive oil 5-10 drops Juniper berry essential oil

Directions:

In a double boiler melt the essential the butter and wax (if any).

Let it cool down to room temperature.

Add the liquid oils, essential oils and the rest of the Ingredients: and stir.

Using a mixer blend at low speed for the first minute and mix well.

Slowly move to high speed until you reach the volume and consistency that you want.

Store in a cool and dry place.

Mandarin And Carrot Seed Body Butter

Ingredients:

1 1/3 cup cocoa butter 2/3 cup jojoba oil 5 drops Carrot Seed essential oil

3 drops Mandarin essential oil

Directions:

In a double boiler melt the essential the butter and wax (if any).

Let it cool down to room temperature.

Add the liquid oils, essential oils and the rest of the Ingredients: and stir.

Using a mixer blend at low speed for the first minute and mix well.

Slowly move to high speed until you reach the volume and consistency that you want.

Store in a cool and dry place.

Cedar Wood And Peanut Body Butter

Ingredients:

1 1/3 cup shea butter 2/3 cup peanut oil 9 drops Cedar wood essential oil

Directions:

In a double boiler melt the essential the butter and wax (if any).

Let it cool down to room temperature.

Add the liquid oils, essential oils and the rest of the Ingredients: and stir.

Using a mixer blend at low speed for the first minute and mix well.

Slowly move to high speed until you reach the volume and consistency that you want.

Store in a cool and dry place.

Chapter 5 Basic Body Butter Recipes

Cool Peppermint Body Butter

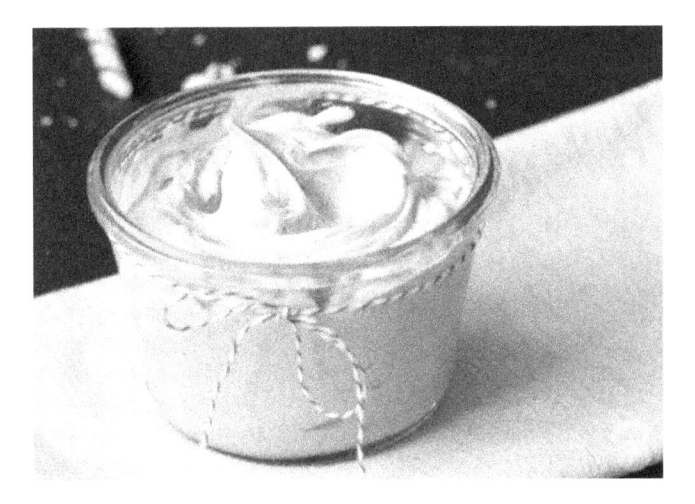

Ingredients:

¼ cup shea butter

¼ cup cocoa butter

¼ cup coconut oil

¼ teaspoon peppermint extract

2 tablespoons vitamin E oil

Directions:

Collect all ingredient expect peppermint into a microwaveable bowl or in a pan place over medium high heat, and heat for about 3 minutes

Stir to ensure any remaining solid pieces have melted. Stir in the peppermint extract.

Transfer to the freezer for few minutes or until the mixture start to solidify but yet still soft.

Transfer to a mixing bowl and whip for six or seven minutes until light and fluffy. You will need to scrape the sides of the bowl occasionally to ensure all is mixed evenly.

Transfer to storage jars and keep in a cool, dark place.

Citrus Body Butter

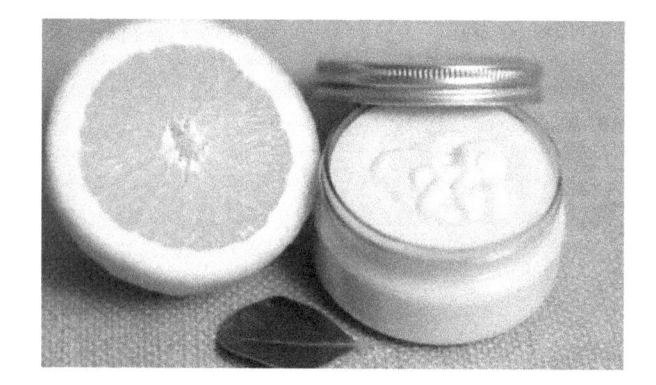

Ingredients:

¼ cup cacao butter

6 tablespoons coconut oil

1 teaspoon lemon essential oil

1 tablespoon vitamin E oil

Directions:

Collect butter and coconut oil in a saucepan and place over low heat until melt and warm.

Remove from heat and add in vitamin E oil and essential oil, stir thoroughly.

Allow to cool at room temperature or until solidified. Store in a cool, dark place.

Nutty Body Butter

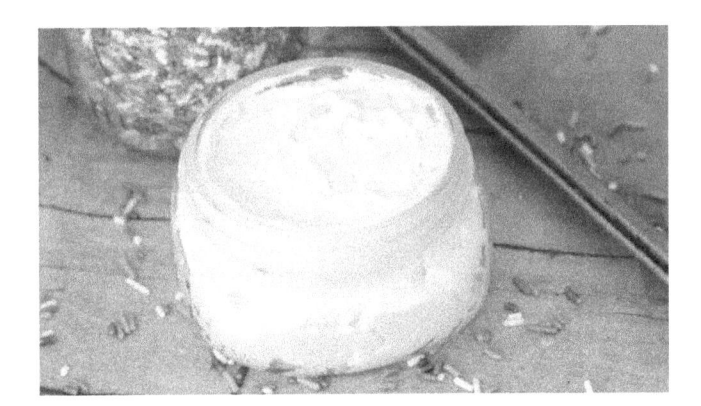

Ingredients:

2 ounces cocoa butter

2 ounces shea butter

2 ounces monoi butter

3 teaspoons aloe vera gel

¼ teaspoon vitamin E oil

3 teaspoons sweet almond oil

1 teaspoon argan oil

10 drops exotic coconut fragrance oil

Directions:

Collect together cocoa butter, shea butter and monoi butters in a pan, place over medium low heat, for few seconds or until melt. Keep heating for 20 more minutes, do not allow to boil.

Add all the remaining ingredients and stir thoroughly.

Pour into a large bowl and cover before allowing to stand overnight. Whip with a hand mixer until fluffy.

Place in storage jars and keep in a cool, dark place.

Berries Body Butter

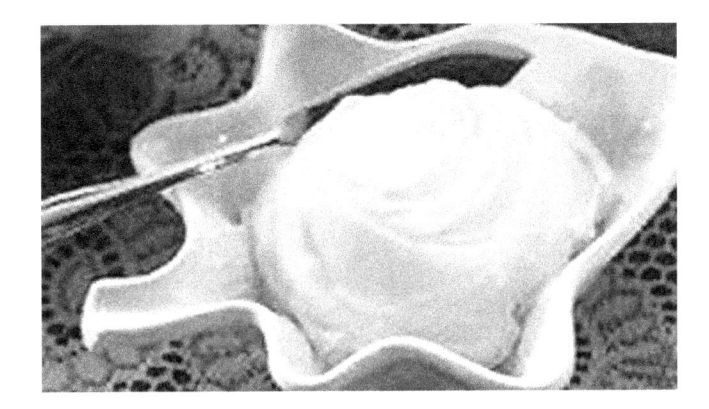

Ingredients:

1 tablespoon frozen cranberries

1 tablespoon shea butter

¼ cup coconut oil

1 drop orange essential oil

Directions:

Collect shea butter and coconut oil together in a medium size mixing bowl and mix well for 5 – 8 minutes.

Put frozen cranberries into a blender cup, blend into small pieces. Add cranberries to the oil and butter mixture and sieve through a fine mesh using a spatula.

Add oil and mix with a spoon. Transfer to container and keep the in the fridge.

SKIN CARE

Beeswax Body Butter

Ingredients:

½ cup coconut oil

½ cup beeswax

1 cup extra virgin olive oil

20 drops lemon essential oil

Directions:

Collect all ingredient expect essential oil in a jar of a least one pint. Heat an inches of water in a saucepan large enough to contain the jar is now placed over medium heat.

Cover the top of the jar (loosely) and pop into the pan of water. When thoroughly melted and mixed allow to cool, at room temperature add your choice of essential oil.

Stir every 10 – 20 minutes to prevent separation before it solidifies.

Tropical Body Butter

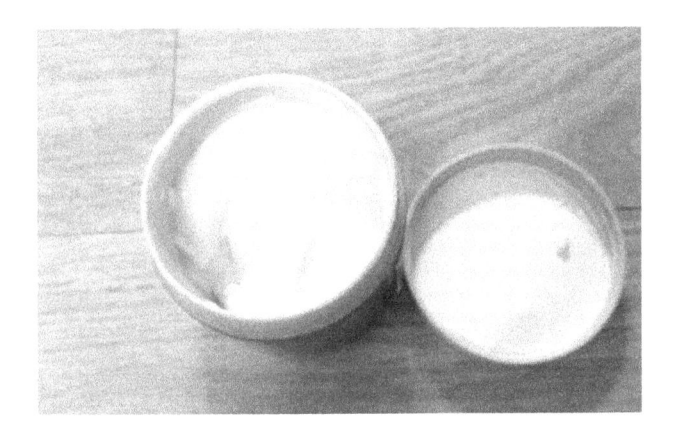

Ingredients:

¼ cup apricot kernel oil

¾ a cup mango butter

1 teaspoon fragrance oil of your choice

Directions:

Collect all ingredients in a microwaveable bowl or pan. Heat over low setting for few seconds, just to soften it, not to melt it.

Stir butter well in other to blend, by using mixer for about 5 minutes, more liquid is from. Place bowl in the freezer for up to ten minutes.

Remove from freezer and blend the mixture for few second. Return bowl to freezer again for another 5 minutes. remove from freezer and blend again for about make sure is well blend.

Repeat all this process several times until you find the mixture to be the consistency of whipped cream. Take care not to overly melt or freeze the mixture.

Anti Bacterial Body Butter

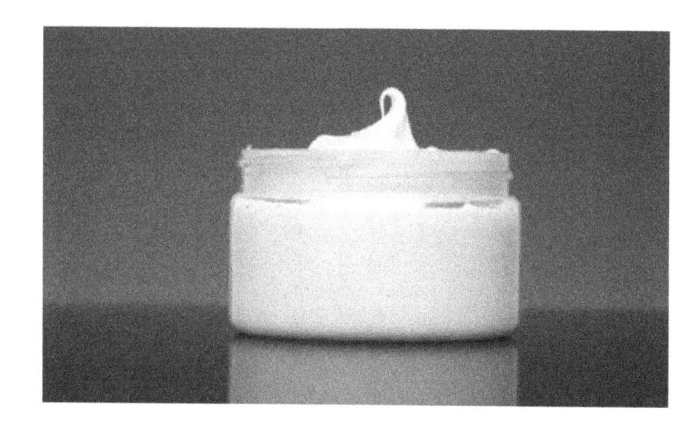

Ingredients:

6 tablespoons cocoa butter   2 tablespoons sesame oil

½ cup of coconut oil   15 drops (or more) of tea tree oil

Your favorite essential oil to mask the tea tree oil scent

Directions:

Collect cocoa butter into a container, place over medium low heat, make sure it does not get too hot, but just enough to melt the solid butter.

Once melted, remove from heat and add sesame and coconut oil, stir well and allow to solidify either in room temperature or by hastening the process through the use of your freezer.

Once firm, whip well by using a mixer for a few minutes. If it does not whip well, you can bring it back to the fridge, allowing it to harden once more.

Add the tea tree oil before mixing it one last time. Keep this in a sanitized and airtight container. Leaving it in the fridge lengthens its shelf life.

Rose Body Butter

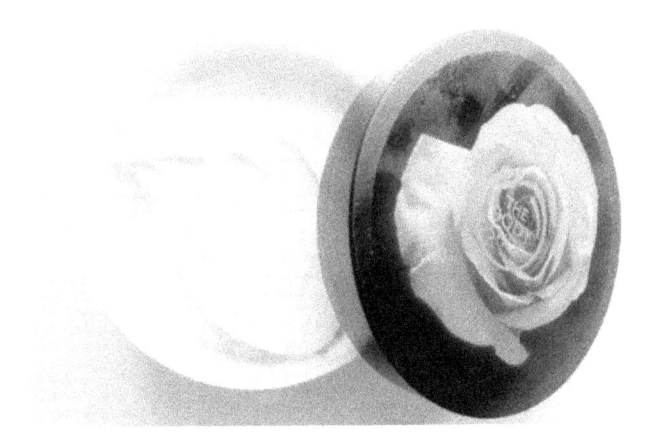

Ingredients:

3 grams cornstarch   10 drops sesame oil   60 grams refined coconut oil

10 grams jojoba oil 1 teaspoon alkanet infused oil

10 drops rose essential oil

Directions:

Take a glass bowl and in it, mix all of your oils except for the rose one. Add the cornstarch and heat it over a pan of simmering water or using a double boiler. Wait until everything is mixed together.

Allow this to cool at room temp so it can set slowly.

Once it's cooled down, add your rose essential oil and whip until it resembles frosting. It needs to be light but firm and fluffy.

Spoon it into a sanitized jar. This is best refrigerated.

Lavender Infused Body Butter

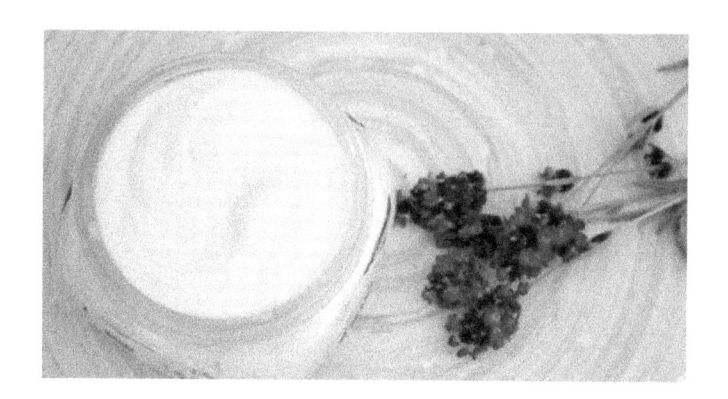

Ingredients:

2 tablespoon beeswax

½ tablespoon olive oil

4 tablespoon coconut oil

3 tablespoons aloe vera gel

1 tablespoon sesame oil

1 teaspoon honey

2 teaspoons lanolin

1 vitamin E capsule

10 drops lavender essential oil

Directions:

Collect oil together with beeswax and honey in a container, heat over medium low heat for few seconds or until melt.

Heat aloe in a pan, place over medium low heat, until melt Once melt, add your beeswax mixture and stir until it well mixes together well.

Add in your lanolin and stir again. Once everything has incorporated properly, turn your heat even lower and add your essential oil along with the vitamin E.

Allow to cool down for about 30 minutes or more depending on the need. Whip it until it becomes smooth.

Transfer to a small jar and allow to cool before covering.

Mint Infused Coconut Body Butter

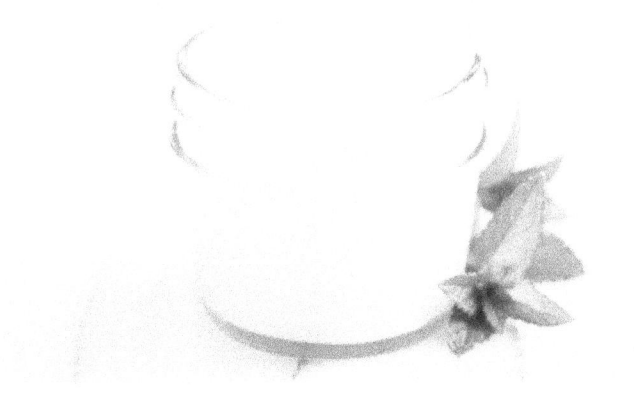

Ingredients:

1 tablespoon mint infused coconut oil

1 tablespoon olive oil

dried rose petals or fresh rosemary

2 tablespoons solid shea butter

1 ml vitamin E or 1 capsule

7 drops lime or lavender essential oil

Directions:

Collect coconut oil and shea butter in a continer, place over medium low heat, for few seconds or until melt.

Add in the herbs, if use. If you are adding the rosemary or rose petals, make sure to heat this mixture for about 30 minutes.

Strain it carefully after and squeeze the oil out from the herbs. Wait until your mixture gets cooler before adding your vitamin E and the essential oils you have chosen.

Whip until it gets fluffy and think. This should take about 5 – 10 minutes. You can let it cool for longer to make the whipping much easier.

Transfer it to a sanitized jar and you're done.

Magnesium Body Butter With Coconut Oil

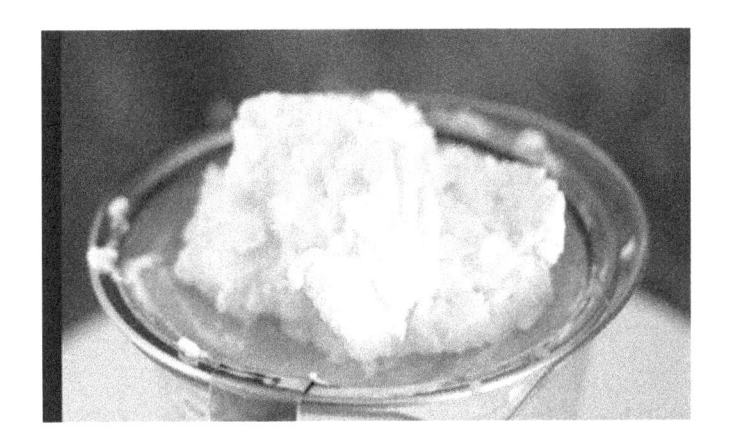

Ingredients:

2 tablespoons beeswax pastilles   ½ cup magnesium flakes

¼ cup unrefined coconut oil   3 tablespoons boiling water

3 tablespoons shea butter

Directions:

Collect magnesium flakes and boiling water together. in a small container, Stir well until it dissolves completely. Think liquid is form, set aside and allow to cool.

Take a mason jar or anything similar and place it in a small pan containing half an inch of water. In the jar, combine your beeswax, coconut oil and Shea butter. Keep your heat on medium.

Once melted properly, remove your jar from the pan very carefully as it could be really hot. Allow to cool in room temperature. The mixture itself should turn slightly opaque.

Transfer into a blender cup, blend at medium speed, whip well.

While blending, slowly add your dissolved magnesium bit by bit to the mixture. Keep blending until everything is well incorporated.

Transfer to the fridge to firm for about 15 minutes. return back to the blender, blend until you get the consistency that you want.

Store in a sanitized container and to keep longer, store it in the fridge.

White Chocolate Peppermint Body Butter

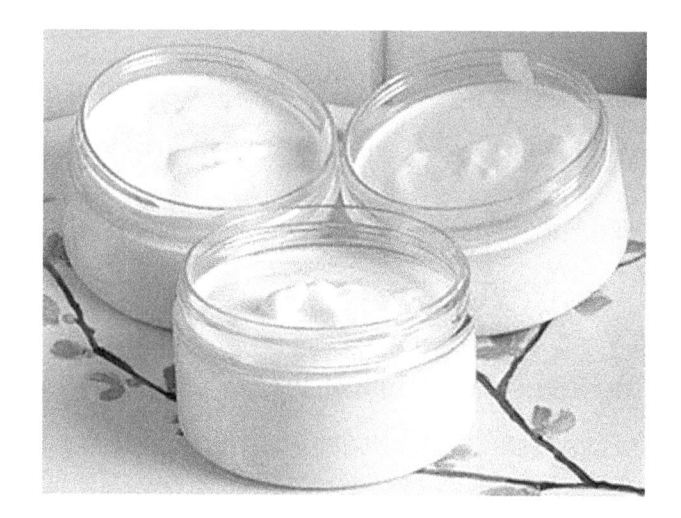

Ingredients:

¼ cup coconut oil

¼ cup cocoa butter

1/8 cup avocado oil

1 teaspoon red raspberry seed oil

10 drops peppermint essential oil

Directions:

Melt butter, avocado oil and coconut oil, in saucepan over low heat. Make sure it does not get really hot. Just enough warm to melt the mixture.

Remove from heat and allow to cool for about 5 minutes. Add raspberry seed oil mix and transfer to freezer or fridge. Allow it to cool for about 60 minutes or until firm enough to be whipped. Even if there is some liquid left, a small amount of it should be fine.

Remove from fridge and add your essential oil.

Whip it for a few minutes until it reaches the desired consistency, firm but not too much. If it does not whip well, just return it to fridge and allow to cool for little more time.

Chapter 6 Body Butter Recipes for Specific Purposes

Wake Me Up Sweet Orange Body Butter

The citrusy aroma of lemon and orange combined is so refreshing — it almost instantaneously wakes you up and fills you with energy. Use it after your morning shower to get that extra boost of energy and kick start your day.

Ingredients:

Shea butter: one cup

Sweet almond oil: half cup

Coconut oil: half cup

Sweet orange essential oil: twenty drops

Lemon essential oil: ten drops

Directions:

Melt the shea butter in a pan using the double boiler method.

Now, add the coconut oil and stir continuously, allowing it to blend.

Remove from heat and place this mixture at room temperature for thirty minutes.

Add the sweet almond oil, sweet orange essential oil and lemon essential oil once the mixture cools down.

Stir properly and place this mixture in the refrigerator for around two hours.

Start whipping the body butter once it achieves a semi solid consistency.

Whip till it peaks and attains a buttery consistency.

Transfer in a glass jar and enjoy how lemon and orange work their magic on your skin.

Magic Of Magnesium Body Butter

Yes, magnesium is truly magical as it helps in absorption of vitamin D. It is great on sore muscles and can be safely used on kids owing to its all-natural Ingredients:. It also helps in nourishing the skin for a softer and silkier you!

Ingredients:

Coconut oil: half cup

Beeswax: four tablespoons

Shea butter: ¼ cup

Natural magnesium flakes: ½ cup

Directions:

Take the magnesium flakes in a small container and pour around three tablespoons of boiling water over them.

Keep stirring until it dissolves, and a thick liquid is formed. Set it aside to cool!

Take the coconut oil, shea butter and beeswax in a separate pan and using the double boiler method, heat on low flame until they melt and blend.

Once they are blended, take the mixture off the flame and allow it to cool.

Pour the magnesium liquid into this mixture once it cools down and whip with a hand blender.

Whip for around ten minutes and then store in the refrigerator to cool down.

Whip once again as the mixture achieves a semi solid consistency.

Continue to whip till you notice a butter like consistency.

Pour into a glass jar, seal with a lid and store in a cool, dry place.

A small batch can keep up to three months without a problem.

Magnetic Mango Body Butter

The high number of antioxidants in mango facilitate clearing and softening of skin, eliminating blackheads and blemishes and cleaning clogged pores. It cools your body and imparts a healthy glow to your skin. The fruity aroma makes you keep coming back for more. No wonder, it is called magnetic!

Ingredients:

Coconut oil: one cup

Shea butter: half cup

Mango butter: half cup

Mango essential oil: thirty drops

Directions:

In a pan, gently melt the coconut oil and shea butter on a very slow flame, using the double boiler method.

When the mixture blends, slowly add the mango butter and blend it for around a minute.

Turn off the heat after a minute and allow it to set for approximately twenty minutes.

When it cools slightly, add thirty drops of mango essential oil into the mixture.

Leave it at room temperature for around twelve hours.

It should appear semi solid by now.

Whip the mixture until it turns fluffy and light.

Place into an airtight glass jar.

Pamper your skin with the magnetic fruity fragrance of mango and nourishment of coconut oil and shea butter. Isn't it heavenly?

Luscious Lavender Body Butter

Relaxing, rejuvenating, calming — these are the words that describe the luscious lavender body butter. Want to treat your sunburns? Go for this completely nourishing and cooling package to give you an ultimate doze of rejuvenation.

Ingredients:

Coconut oil: one cup

Olive oil: ¼ cup

Beeswax: ½ cup

Honey: ¼ cup

Aloe vera gel: four tablespoons

Lanolin: two tablespoons

Lavender essential oil: twenty-five drops

Vitamin E: one capsule

Directions:

In a pan, gently melt the coconut oil, olive oil, beeswax and honey on a very slow flame, using the double boiler method.

In a separate pan, using the same double boiler method heat aloe vera. Mix it with the beeswax mixture once it melts. Continue to stir.

Mix in the lanolin and stir gently.

When everything has blended, turn off the heat and add vitamin E and the lavender essential oil.

Whip with a hand blender until it is smooth, light and fluffy.

Pour into small glass jars and allow it to cool before using. Now, that's what we call simplicity in a bottle!

Magical Citrusy Mango Body Butter

True to its name, this body butter is a little citrusy and a little mango-ish! Truly magical on your skin, this one is a great nourisher and the fruity fragrance ensures that you make a second batch!

Ingredients:

Beeswax: ¼ cup

Cocoa butter: ¾ cup

Shea butter: ¾ cup

Mango butter: one cup

Almond oil: four tablespoons

Vitamin E: two capsules

Sweet orange essential oil: ten drops

Lime essential oil: ten drops

Lemon essential oil: twenty drops

Directions:

In a pan, gently melt the cocoa butter, beeswax, shea butter and mango butter over slow-medium flame, using the double boiler method. Let the mixture stay on the flame for around twenty minutes so that it blends nicely and does not go grainy on cooling. Don't forget to stir consistently.

Stir in the almond oil and vitamin E and remove from heat.

Add the essential oils and stir well, ensuring that everything blends well.

Allow the mixture to cool and set in glass jars.

Voila, ready to use citrusy mango body butter and that too without any whipping!

This one may need a little massage and still leave a little oily feel on the skin, so it is best for use at night. Trust me, you will wake up to a more fresh, supple and satin smooth skin.

Pamper With Pink Body Butter

True to its name, this body butter is a little citrusy and a little mango-ish! Truly magical on your skin, this one is a great nourisher and the fruity fragrance ensures that you make a second batch! Ingredients:

Coconut oil: one cup

Jojoba oil: four tablespoons

Shea butter: ½ cup

Cornstarch: around four grams

Rose essential oil: twenty drops

Directions:

In a pan, gently melt the coconut oil, jojoba oil, shea butter and corn starch over slow-medium heat, using a double boiler method.

Stir continuously until everything mixes well and blends.

Remove from heat and cool for around thirty minutes.

Stir in the rose essential oil and mix well.

Allow the mixture to set in the fridge for around two hours or till it reaches a semi solid consistency.

Remove from the fridge and whip with a hand blender till the mixture becomes light and fluffy. It will start resembling a frosting on the cake.

Spoon out into glass jars and begin the process of pampering your body.

Consume within three months.

Protective Mint Rosemary Shea Body Butter

This luxuriously whipped nourishing and moisturizing creation instantly infiltrates your skin and provides the ultimate protection. I recommend the use of Kukui Nut Oil owing to its high permeability and calming properties. Feel free to substitute with any other oil of your choice if you like. The kukui nut oil can nourish and treat chapped skin due to the presence of a high quantity of essential fatty acids: linoleic and alpha-linolenic acid. This body butter is great to treat dry skin, eczema or psoriasis. Great for sensitive skin too! The mint in the butter provides that great aroma! Truly a delight for the skin!

Ingredients:

Cocoa butter: ½ cup

Shea butter: one cup

Kukui nut oil: ½ cup

Spearmint essential oil: thirty drops

Rosemary essential oil: fifteen drops

Directions:

In a pan, gently melt the cocoa butter, shea butter and kukui nut oil over a slow medium flame, using the double boiler method.

Continue to stir consistently until the oils blend. This will take around eight minutes.

Let the mixture cool up to room temperature for around twenty minutes and then transfer to a freezer for approximately thirty minutes.

Next, blend this mixture with you hand blender for around ten minutes and place it back into the freezer for fifteen minutes.

Whisk once again till you get a butter like consistency and keep it back in the freezer for ten minutes.

Mix the spearmint and rosemary essential oils and whisk once again till the mixture forms a peak.

Store in a cool, dry place and use within sixty days.

You do love you luscious looking skin, don't you?

Chapter 7 Complicated Body Butter Recipes

Homemade Body Butter With Jojoba Oil

With rich shea and cacao butters, this 4-ingredient body butter keeps the skin soft and smooth through even the driest of winters.

Ingredients: ⅓ cup cacao butter* ⅓ cup shea butter ⅓ cup jojoba oil

15-20 drops essential oils**

Directions:

Create a double boiler on the stove by filling a small saucepan halfway with water and placing a glass bowl in the opening of the pan (the bottom of the bowl should not touch the water). Add the cacao butter and the shea butter to the bowl and heat the double boiler over medium heat until the butter is melted. Remove the bowl from the saucepan and add the jojoba oil. At this point, you can mix in any essential oils you want.

Set the bowl in the fridge to chill for about 60 minutes.

When the butter becomes opaque and is set, remove the bowl from the fridge and use the hand mixer or electric mixer to whip the body butter until it's fluffy, about 2-3 minutes.

Scoop the body butter into an airtight container and store it at room temperature, away from light, for up to 6 months.

Diy Frankincense Body Butter

This lovely creamy & smooth body butter smells so good you will want to eat it! And it contains powerful ingredients that support healthy skin!

Frankincense essential oil has been shown to reverse signs of aging, scars and stretchmarks, and treat dry skin.

One of the main benefits of Myrrh essential oil is that it helps to maintain healthy skin. It also soothes cracked skin, and is often added to lotions to relieve skin infections like eczema, acne, ringworm and athlete's foot.

Ingredients: 1/4 cup coconut oil   1/4 cup olive oil

1/4 cup shea butter   1/4 cup beeswax

25 drops of frankincense essential oil 25 drops of myrrh essential oil

Directions:

Place all Ingredients: except the frankincense and myrrh essential oils in a glass bowl over a pot with boiling water on the stove top.

Once all the Ingredients are melted and mixed, take off the stove, allow to cool slightly and put in the refrigerator for 45 minutes.

After 45 minutes, remove from refrigerator and mix with a hand blender until it is creamy and fluffy.

Add the essential oils and mix well with a spoon.

Store in a glass jar. Also lovely to put in a small jar and keep in your handbag as a hand cream or lip moisturizer.

Diy Natural Nipple Butter

What better way to ensure that your nipple cream is all-natural and safe for baby than to make it yourself? And if you're reading this and you aren't a new mom, chances are you know someone who is... and this would be a great and incredibly appreciated DIY gift!

Ingreadients: 1/4 cup Calendula 1/4 cup Marshmallow Root

1 cup Olive oil and/or Coconut oil 1/8 cup Beeswax

2 tbsp Baraka Shea Butter

Directions:

Scoop herbs into a glass jar and pour oil on top. Make sure there is at least one inch gap between the mixture and top of the jar. Screw lid on tightly. Set out a medium size slow cooker and line the bottom with a thick hand towel. Place the jar inside and fill the slow cooker with water up to the level of the oil in the jar, but keep the water level below the lid. Turn the slow cooker on the "warm" setting and leave it on for 3 to 5 days, partially covered. Add more water into the cooker when necessary. After 3 to 5 days, remove the oil infusion from the cooker and let it fresh, a little. Strain the oil through a fine sieve and cheesecloth into a small stainless steel sauce pan. Squeeze with your hands or use the back of a spoon to release the finished oil. Throw the used herbs away. Add beeswax and shea butter into the sauce pan and turn heat on low. Stir until wax and butter has melted. Pour the mixture into glass jars or tins. Allow them to cool completely before putting the lids on. Date and label the nipple cream. Keep them in a cool, dry and dark spot. Will keep for several months.

DIY 'Make Me Shine' And 'Bronze Me Beautiful'

Sometimes we all need a little extra magic, right? This shimmering whipped body butter is packed with a multicolored blend of pearlescent mica and iridescent glitter. Its fluffy whipped texture allows the butter to glide onto the skin, leaving it feeling soft, supple, and coated with sparkles.

Ingredients:

40 grams deodorized cocoa butter 30 grams watermelon seed oil

20 grams virgin coconut oil 10 grams candelilla wax

5 grams lavender glow mica 2 grams superfine silk powder

2.5 ml cardamom & primrose plant-based fragrance oil

2 grams cosmetic glitter (optional)

Directions:

Combine cocoa butter and candelilla wax in double boiler and heat until melted. Add virgin coconut oil and watermelon seed oil. Stir until melted, then remove pot from heat. Add mica, silk powder, and glitter, then whisk until well blended.

Fill a mixing bowl or sauce pan with cold water and place double boiler inside. Whisk mixture vigorously as it cools and thickens.

When mixture begins to thicken, add plant-based fragrance oil. Continue to whisk until body butter becomes thick and fluffy.

Transfer to jars and cool until stiff.

Homemade Herbal Infused Whipped Body Butter

Make an herbal infused body butter using calendula, chamomile, lavender and marshmallow root. These herbs are infused with jojoba oil and avocado oil to create moisturizing and soothing body butter for softening and soothing dry, cracked hands and skin.

Ingredients:

1/2 tbsp Calendula

1/2 tbsp Chamomile

1/2 tbsp Lavender

1/2 tbsp Marshmallow Root

1/4 cup Shea Butter

1/4 cup Cocoa Butter

1/4 cup Jojoba Oil

1/4 cup Avocado Oil

Optional: Essential Oils – I personally don't use them in this recipe.

Optional: 1 tsp non-gmo Vitamin E oil

Optional: Arrowroot Powder

Directions:

In a double boiler combine the herbs with Jojoba Oil and Avocado Oil.

Bring to a boil, then turn the burner to low and allow the herbs and allow to infuse for at least 2 hours.

In a separate pan combine the Shea butter and Cocoa butter over low heat. Once melted, remove from the heat.

Using a strainer, strain the herbs from the Jojoba and Avocado oil infusion.

In a mixing bowl combine the Shea/Cocoa butter and the Jojoba/Avocado oils. Then place bowl in the refrigerator until the oils have thickened.

Use a mixer to whip the butter and oils until you get a creamy, thick consistency.

If you don't get the right consistency at first, stick the mixture back in the fridge to cool more and then mix again with the mixer.

Place body butter into a jar and cover with a lid.

Diy Hemp Oil Body Butter

Homemade skin-care products are a wonderful way to create a product tailored to your specific needs. We're big fans of body butters, so we decided to adapt this Rosemary Citrus Body Balm recipe by Home Song blog to include our favorite plant, cannabis.

Ingredients:

1/2 c. coconut oil (moisturizing, antifungal, antiviral) or if using a LEVO - 1/2 c. herbal infused coconut oil (we used lavender & rosemary!)

1/2 c shea butter

1/4 c. hemp oil

1/4 c. beeswax pellets

approximately 2 glass jars, depending on size

essential oils (approximately 30 drops total)

Directions:

To infuse your coconut oil: Add 1/2 c coconut oil to LEVO basin & fill pod with lavender & rosemary. Infuse at 200°F for 30 min. Remove pod; note that it will be hot!

To make your body butter: Add shea butter, beeswax pellets, and hemp oil then set at 150°F for 15 min.

Add essential oils then immediately dispense to avoid beeswax hardening in basin

Without a LEVO:

Melt coconut oil, shea butter, hemp oil, and beeswax pellets in a double boiler then pour the liquid into glass jars.

Add essential oils and stir until desired aroma is achieved. We started with 5 drops of each essential oil, then increased from there.

Diy Pomegranate Seed Whipped Body Butter

This is a luscious whipped body butter packed full of healthy nutrients that will leave your skin feeling moisturized and happy!

Ingredients: 4 oz. of Shea Butter 2 oz. of Coconut Oil

1 oz. of Cocoa Butter 1 oz. of Pomegranate Seed Oil 6 Glass jars

Directions:

Using a 16 oz. glass measuring cup in a small pan of water, melt the cocoa butter over low heat until almost liquefied. Add the shea butter and coconut oil until the mixture completely melts. Once these oils are melted together, add the pomegranate seed oil.

Based on your therapeutic and/or energetic intention, choose 2-4 essential oils to incorporate into this blend. Listed below are three example blends just in case you want a few ideas for inspiration!

Using a glass stir rod, gently blend in the essential oils. Then, cover and place this mixture in the refrigerator for about 30-90 minutes until partially cooled. This is a step that can't be rushed. If preferred, place in the freezer for about 20 minutes, checking consistency about every 15 minutes. The blend should be stirrable but not liquid.

Remove cooled oils from the refrigerator. Using a hand-held blender, whip the mixture until it is the desired consistency. It should be beautifully light and fluffy!

Pour into 2 oz. glass jars, and enjoy!

Homemade Toning Coffee Infused Body Butter

This luxurious coffee body butter moisturizes and tones skin! Use it daily on problem areas to reduce the appernce of cellulite and uneven skin.

Ingredients:

1/4 cup organic coffee beans   1/2 cup virgin coconut oil

1/2 cup cocoa butter   1/2 cup extra virgin olive oil

Directions:

Melt 1/2 cup of virgin coconut oil in a saucepan on low heat.

Add 1/4 cup of whole organic coffee beans.

Keep the oil on low heat for 20 minutes, stirring occasionally.

Use a fine mesh strainer to strain the coconut toil from the coffee beans.

Melt the cocoa butter in a small saucepan over low heat.

Once the cocoa butter is melted, add olive oil and coffee infused coconut oil. Remove from heat.

Refrigerate the oils for 25-30 minutes, or until the oils just begin to solidify.

Use a hand mixer or stand mixer to whip the oils into butter. This will take 10-15 minutes to achieve a soft and fluffy texture.

Scoop the coffee body butter into a storage container and store in a cool dry place. Use daily on dry or problem areas.

SKIN CARE

Chapter 8 Body Butter Recipes for Different Kinds of Skin

Anti-Ageing Body Butter

Ingredients:

1 cup raw shea butter   1 cup raw coconut oil   ¼ cup almond oil

½ teaspoon Vitamin E oil or 2-3 Vitamin E capsules

20-40 drops of essential oils of your choice (optional)

Directions:

Do you dream about soft, beautiful skin? Do not worry because this anti-aging body butter gets you covered. Shea butter minimizes stretch marks and restores skin's elasticity. Coconut oil is a great moisturizer. Almond oil contains vitamin D & E, known for preventing premature skin ageing and promoting healthy skin. Melt shea butter and coconut oil in a double boiler over medium heat. This should take about 15 minutes. Allow the melted mixture to cool before adding vitamin E, essential oils (if any) and almond oil. Then chill it in a fridge for half an hour until it turns semi-solid. Next, you may want to whisk it with a hand mixer until it gets light fluffy consistence. The body butter is ready! This butter will give your skin very nice, soft feel; it is not too greasy, and it does not block the skin pores. Just apply a bit and you will not have to wait long for results.

Anti-Bacterial Body Butter

Ingredients:

½ cup coconut oil

6 tablespoons cocoa butter

2 tablespoons jojoba oil

15-20 drops tea tree oil

Directions:

This body butter is a genuinely versatile all-in-one skincare product – a moisturiser, an anti-bacterial treatment; it can be used as after-shave cream on legs and underarms, or as a natural deodorant!

For this recipe, you will need coconut oil, cocoa butter, jojoba oil and tea tree essential oil.

Melt cocoa butter in a double boiler over low temperature. It should be dissolved not hot! Once it's melted, remove it from the heat and allow it to cool for 10 minutes before adding jojoba oil and coconut oil. Wait for some hours or leave it overnight so that the mixture solidifies in room temperature. Alternatively, you can speed up this process using a fridge. Once the blend gets solid, whisk is using a hand mixer. Add in tea tree oil and mixt it one last time. Apply on clean skin, especially on over dried areas, like heels, elbows, calves.

Tea tree oil is great for a range of skin problem, like acne, dermatitis, psoriasis, and does not require an introduction. It efficiently kills bacteria, fungi and even some viruses and neutralizes bad skin odour.

Skin Perfecting Body Butter

Ingredients:

2 oz. shea butter

2 oz. evening primrose oil

10 drops jasmine oil

10 drops Frankincense Oil

Directions:

Are you after beautiful and soft skin? If so, then try this anti-scars and anti-stretch marks body butter. You will need shea butter, evening primrose oil, jasmine oil and frankincense oil. It is a perfect combination: evening primrose oil increases skin's flexibility and hydration, jasmine oil helps fade dark spots and scars, while frankincense oil reduces the appearance of stretch marks.

Melt shea butter in a double boiler. When it becomes liquefied (but not hot!) add evening primrose oil and mix these two Ingredients: with a hand or electric mixer. Pour the blend into a container and place in a fridge until it gets cool, but not solid. It usually takes a couple of minutes only. Then remove it from the fridge, stir in jasmine and frankincense oils and whip it with a mixer until light and creamy. Pour into containers and let the butter cool before applying onto the skin.

You can use this body butter safely on stretch marks, burns, scars, broken skin, knees, elbows, hands, even on lips. It smells and feels amazing!

Need & Turmeric Body Butter

Ingredients:

50g coconut oil

1lbs olive oil

30g beeswax   3 tablespoons turmeric juice

10 neem leaves   10 holy holy basil leaves

5 capsules Vitamin E

5-10 drops essential oil of your choice

Directions:

To make this butter, pour coconut oil in a clean pan and put in neem and holy basil leaves. Let it boil for a couple of minutes, then remove from the heat and put aside to cool down. Then, strain the oil.

Next, heat gently coconut oil, olive oil and almond oil in a double boiler. Stir in turmeric juice. The mixture will be giving crackling sound; this is normal and nothing to be worry about. Next, add beeswax and keep stirring until it gets completely melted. Squeeze vitamin E into the mixture. You may want now to add essential oils of your choice, such as ylang ylang, or rosemary. Pour the mixture into a clean container and leave it for a couple of hours to cool and set up.

In Asian cultures turmeric and other species are commonly used in skincare

Rich Cocoa Body Butter

Ingredients:

3 oz. coca butter

1 oz. Vitamin E oil

1 tablespoon unsweetened cocoa powder

5-10 drops vanilla essential oil

Directions:

Cocoa butter and shea butter are similar in many aspects: they are both natural powerful skin moisturisers, rich in fatty acids. They are both effective in treatment of eczema, psoriasis and other skin ailments. However, some people find shea butter's fragrance unappealing, or even off-putting. In contrast, most users agree that the smell of cocoa butter is very pleasant and can enhance the mood. This body butter is a great treat for all cocoa butter fans.

Heat cocoa butter over low heat in a double boiler. Once it gets completely melted, add cocoa powder and vitamin E, stirring. Next, add 10-15 drops of vanilla essential oils. Then blend off the heat, pour into a clean container and leave aside to cool down. Cocoa butter gives the mixture the fragrance of rich chocolate. Hmmm…..Yummy Don't get tempted to eat

Royal Body Butter

Ingredients:

4 tablespoon coconut oil 1-2 tablespoon olive oil 2 tablespoon beeswax

1 tablespoon honey 3 tablespoon aloe vera gel 2 tablespoon lanolin

1 Vitamin E capsule

10 drops lavender essential oil

Directions

This body butter is based on a royal combination of honey, aloe vera, vitamin E and lavender, the most appreciated Ingredients: applied in natural skincare.

Aloe vera is used in most expensive skincare products and does not really require an introduction. It contains a range of antioxidants, such as: vitamin C and E, or beta carotene, helping the skin to maintain its natural firmness and keeps it well-hydrated. Aloe vera reduces visibility of stretch marks and stimulates the growth of new skin cells.

Place oils, honey and beeswax in a double boiler and melt them over low heat, stirring. Once all the Ingredients: get melted, add aloe vera and lanolin to the mixture. Stir in vitamin E and lavender essential oils. Remove the mixture from the heat and let it cool. If you prefer lighter texture, you can whisk the butter with a hand mixer until fluffy. The butter is ready. Apply and enjoy!

Whipped Kokum Body Butter

Ingredients:

20 g kokum butter

10 g sweet almond oil

10-15 drops essential oils of your choice

Directions:

This recipe, instead of popular shea, cocoa or mango butter, uses much less known kokum butter. Kokum butter originates from India, where it first got recognition for its high fatty acids content. The butter is well known for its strong regenerative properties, making it a perfect treatment for damaged skin. Is it really so good? You can check for yourself.

This is one of the easiest body butter recipes. All you need to do is to measure and place the butter and sweet almond oil in a double boiler and heat them slowly until fully melted. Then, add essential oils of your choice and stir well. Take the mixture off the heat and leave it aside to chill. Whip the butter with a hand, or electric mixer until light and fluffy. Apply on clean skin.

Cupuacu Whipped Body Butter

Ingredients:

¾ cup shea butter

¾ cup cupuacu butter

5 oz. olive oil (or sunflower oil)

8 drops Vitamin E oil (optional)

20 drops essential oils of your choice

Directions:

Have you ever heard of cupuacu butter? It originates from the Rain Forest and contains a high level of polyphenols, which combat free radicals and fatty acids to moisture and protect the skin. It is also known for absorbing UVA rays (natural sun protection).

To make this body butter, melt cocoa butter and cupuacu butter in a double boiler. Remove from the heat as soon as they get melted. Next, add olive oil, vitamin E and essential oils (lavender, rose geranium, sweet orange are nice) and mix well. Pour the mixture into a clean container and let it cool, then whip with a mixer.

Apply on clean skin after a shower, or just anytime. Massage some extra onto hands, feet, cracked heals or elbows. This body butter can be also applied on coarse hair.

Shea & Kukui Body Butter

Ingredients:

¼ cup cocoa butter

1 cup shea butter 2 tablespoons kukui oil

1 tablespoon rosehip or Sea Buckthorn oil

1 capsule Vitamin E oil (optional)

1 teaspoon corn starch (optional)

Directions:

This body butter is different from all others, as it uses kukui oil as carrier oil, a great natural skincare ingredient.

The kukui tree itself is probably the most known as the state tree of Hawaii. The oil is pressed from the seeds (nuts) of the tree and is used in many different ways: as natural sun protection, skin healer, hair conditioner, etc. It contains high level of fatty acids, which are essential for healthy, young looking skin. It is also rich in vitamins A, E and C, protecting the skin from free radicals and environmental stress. If you can get hold of kukui oil, do not hesitate and make this wonderful body butter!

Place cocoa and shea butter is a double boiler and let it melt slowly, but do not allow to boil or even simmer. Once the butters have melted, remove the pot from the heat and add the remaining Ingredients: and mix well. Let the butter aside to chill. Once it is cool, whisk it with a mixer until it looks like whipped cream.

Body Butter For Extra Dry Skin

Ingredients:

2 ½ tablespoons cocoa butter

1 tablespoon coconut oil

2 tablespoons sweet almond oil

1 tablespoon sesame oil

1 tablespoon grated beeswax

Directions:

No matter how hard you try to get your skin ready for winter, cold temperatures and winds can make it dry and flaky. This is where this body butter comes handy. It is based on the combination of super-rich and easy to access Ingredients: which can make your skin glow even in the most severe weather!

You will need cocoa butter, coconut oil, sweet almond oil, sesame oil and some beeswax. They are all excellent moisturisers, skin softeners and healers. Cocoa butter smells delicious already, so you don't really need to add any fragrances. Beeswax will also add some subtle scent of honey.

Choose high quality beeswax for your butter….

Once you got all the Ingredients: ready, place them in a double boiler and heat slowly until all melted. Next, remove the mixture from the heat and let it cool in a room temperature or you can use a fridge to speed up the process.

When the mix become solid, transfer the butter to a clean container as use often as you need – there is no rights and wrongs with this butter.

Chapter 9 More Complicated Body Butter Recipes and Regimens

Goat Milk Body Butter

Makes: 4 ounces time: 20 minutes

Good for: all skin types

This body butter is easy to use and travels well. It provides your skin with long-lasting moisture. The goat milk makes your skin feel smooth, soft, and silky, while the essential fatty acids boost its moisture content.

Ingredients:

2 tablespoons beeswax

2 tablespoons apricot oil

1 tablespoon castor oil

2 tablespoons avocado oil

1 tablespoon goat milk

Directions:

In a mini slow cooker or double boiler that you've dedicated to beeswax products, melt the beeswax.

Once the beeswax is melted, add everything except the goat milk. Stir with a spoon or mini whisk that you've dedicated to beeswax products. When the oils and beeswax are completely incorporated and melted, turn the heat off, add the goat milk, and stir. Remember to add goat milk that's been warmed. See here for more about beeswax.

Transfer to a low-profile jar for ease of use. Be mindful that the product will be hot, so make sure you pour it into a container that can withstand the heat. Silicone molds work perfectly. Use a mold capacity that will work well for you to hold and apply. I like disc shapes for body butters.

TO USE: Apply onto your body where desired.

STORAGE: Store in a cool, dry place for 4–8 months.

USE: As needed

DID YOU KNOW?

Low-profile jars are ideal for storing your body butters. The wider mouth and shorter stature make it easier to get the product out. If you use a mold, the butter will be loose so you can hold it and apply it directly on your skin for ease of application. After use, you can replace the molded butter into a container for storage.

Coconut Body Butter

Makes: about 4 ounces time: 30 minutes

Good for: all skin types

Coconut is a multitasking skin-care ingredient. That's why you'll often see it included in skin-care products. This body butter has both the active properties of the coconut's milk and meat, giving it everything from a rounded essential fatty acid profile to antibacterial and antifungal properties. It's great for the whole body, but it's an especially wonderful treat for your feet!

Ingredients:

2 tablespoons beeswax

2 tablespoons coconut oil

1 tablespoon castor oil

2 tablespoons coconut butter

1½ tablespoons coconut milk

Directions:

In a mini slow cooker or double boiler that you've dedicated to beeswax products, melt the beeswax.

Once the beeswax is melted, add everything except the coconut milk. Stir with a spoon or mini whisk that you've dedicated to beeswax products. When the oils and beeswax are completely incorporated and melted, turn the heat off, add the coconut milk, and stir. Remember to add the coconut milk that's been is warmed.

Transfer to a low-profile jar for ease of use. Be mindful that the product will be hot, so make sure you pour it into a container that can withstand the heat. Silicone molds work perfectly. Use a mold capacity that will work well for you to hold and apply. I like disc shapes for body butters.

TO USE: Apply onto your body where desired.

STORAGE: Store in a cool, dry place for 3–5 months.

USE: As needed

GIFT IT

For a really special treat, create a coconut-themed gift basket. Stock up on your coconut products to make Coconut Sugar Lip Scrub (here), Coconut Lip Balm (here), and this Coconut Body Butter. Don't forget your decorative jars and labels!

Butter Balm

Makes: about 5 ounces time: 30 minutes

Good for: all skin types

This is a true butter balm. It uses three types of butter, instead of oils mixed with stearic acid (such as "avocado butter" or "olive butter"), to make a butter-like consistency. This recipe is great for extremely dry, cracked skin, so it's a great go-to for those who live in places with harsh winters.

Ingredients:

¼ cup cocoa butter

¼ cup shea butter

1 teaspoon coconut butter

2 tablespoons avocado oil

2 drops any essential oil or a combination (optional)

Directions:

On the stovetop in a small pot, melt the cocoa butter over low heat.

Add coconut butter to the pot and melt on low heat.

Remove from the heat and add the shea butter to the melted cocoa and coconut butters. The heat from the butters should be enough to melt them. If not, return to the lowest setting on the stovetop and stir until melted. Remove from the heat.

Add the avocado oil and essential oils, if using, and mix well.

Transfer to a low-profile jar for ease of use and place in the freezer immediately till completely cooled.

TO USE: Apply onto your body wherever you desire.

STORAGE: Store in a cool, dry place for 3–5 months.

USE: As often as needed

A CLOSER LOOK

When shea butter melts and reconstitutes slowly, it will crystallize, or ball up. To avoid this, make sure you carefully, and slowly, melt the butter over low heat and immediately transfer it to the freezer after mixing in all the other Ingredients:. This rapid cooling gives you a luscious finished product.

SAMPLE WEEKLY REGIMENS

Here you'll find a few sample weekly regimens based on your skin type. (See here for descriptions of skin types.) Try these regimens at the start of your DIY skin-care journey. As you practice more and begin to see results, feel free to change up your routine. Skin actually responds well when you alter your routine at least once a year.

DRY SKIN

MORNING AND EVENING: Wash with Coconut Cleanser (here), follow up with Cucumber Toner (here), and finish with Macadamia, Kukui Nut & Avocado Moisturizer (here). Once daily, while in the shower, apply Goat Milk, Avocado & Honey Mask (here).

TWICE A WEEK: Switch out your mask for Pumpkin, Coconut & Brown Sugar Mask (here).

If skin is persistently dry, add Hydrating Serum (here) after toning, but before moisturizing.

NORMAL SKIN

MORNING AND EVENING: Wash with Strawberry, Honey & Oat Cleanser (here), follow up with Cucumber, Lemon & Tea Toner (here) or, to help smooth out wrinkles, Rose Hip & Citrus Toner (here). Complete your routine with Argan, Carrot & Sesame Moisturizer (here).

ONCE A WEEK, WHILE IN THE SHOWER: Avocado, Yogurt & Brewer's Yeast Mask (here).

COMBINATION SKIN

MORNING AND EVENING: Wash with Honey & Chia Seed Cleanser (here) and follow up with Tea & Vinegar Detox Toner (here). Finish with Argan, Carrot & Sesame Moisturizer (here).

ONCE A WEEK: Dead Sea Mud, Kombucha & Brewer's Yeast Mask (here).

OILY SKIN

MORNING AND EVENING: Wash with Activated Charcoal Cleanser (here) and follow up with Apple Juice, Sparkling Wine & Beer Toner (here) and St. John's Wort, Hemp & Avocado Moisturizer (here).

ONCE OR TWICE A WEEK: While in the shower, apply Turmeric, Yogurt & Honey Mask (here).

MATURE SKIN

MORNING AND EVENING: Wash with Hemp Cleanser (here) and follow up with Rose Hip & Citrus Toner (here). Finish with St. John's Wort, Hemp & Avocado Moisturizer (here).

ONCE OR TWICE A WEEK: While in the shower, apply Paprika, Honey & Buttermilk Mask (here).

Here are a few additional guidelines:

• Be sure to detox your skin at least once a year.

• If you have very oily or dry skin and are not getting the results you want, clean your pores. Do a deep-pore cleaning and use detox products for a month. Also pay close attention to other products you use that come in contact with your face, like shampoo and conditioner. Some OTC brands include Ingredients: that can clog and congest pores.

• If you have blemishes, do not exfoliate unless the recipe indicates it is for blemished skin.

• Start using the anti-aging products at the first signs of wrinkles.

• Skin can change types and needs over the course of your life, so keep up with your skin needs, not your skin image.

MORE INFORMATION ON SEEKING SAFE INGREDIENTS:

It's very important to dig into the labels of any lotions or potions you are thinking of buying or already have on hand. The fronts of beauty bottles are often filled with claims about the product within, but the back is where you can find out if a product is in line with your criteria of what you deem safe and acceptable.

To find out what an ingredient is and if it's harmful, a good resource is the Material Data Safety Sheet (MSDS), which can be found online. This document provides health and safety information about substances, products, and chemicals. This is the same information and guidelines used by chemists when working with or handling these Ingredients: and it is provided to manufacturers and the consumer as well. Below is a list of Ingredients: I try to avoid.

INGREDIENTS: TO AVOID:

- Diethanolamine (DEA)

- Formaldehyde

- Nanoparticles

- Parabens

- Petroleum

- Phthalates

- Propylene glycol

- PVP/VA copolymer

- Synthetic fragrances

- Triethanolamine (TEA)

INGREDIENTS: TO LOOK FOR:

- Arrowroot, in place of talc powder

- Colorants from minerals, to replace synthetic dyes

- Edible Ingredients: from your kitchen (honey, oatmeal, avocado, etc.)

- Essential oils instead of fragrance

- Extracts that list what they are extracted in, such "green tea extracted in organic grape alcohol"

- Fragrance-free products

- Nonfoaming facial cleansers and non-detergent body cleansers

- Powdered products, hard bar lotions that are made without water (which require less preservation and, therefore, fewer chemicals)

- Pure butters, such as shea and coconut

Whipped Shea & Body Oil Butter

Makes: about 4 ounces time: 20 minutes

Good for: all skin types

Pure shea butter is second to none. I like to whip it to make it fluffier, lighter, and easier to apply.

Ingredients: ½ cup unrefined shea butter

⅛ cup Basic Body Oil (here)

5 drops any essential oil or combination (optional)

Directions:

With a hand mixer, beat shea butter on high for 30 seconds. To make the best whipped butter, warm the shea up with your hands (do not heat it). You can take the ½ cup of butter, put it in plastic wrap, and hold it in your closed hands to warm, or with sanitized hands you can hold it till it warms up.

Slowly pour in the Basic Body Oil and essential oils, if using, and continue mixing for 5 minutes until whipped.

Transfer to a low-profile jar for ease of use.

TO USE: Apply onto body where desired.

STORAGE: Store in a cool, dry place for 3–5 months.

USE: As often as needed

A CLOSER LOOK

Many OTC butters aren't made of butter at all. Instead, oils (like olive or avocado oil) or juices (like aloe vera juice) are mixed with stearic acid, which is an emulsifier, to create a substance that resembles butter. Products made with stearic acid aren't necessarily bad for you, but they are not real butters and will not offer the same benefits. Oils and butters have different uses and different properties. When you use the right Ingredients: in the right places, you'll notice a significant change in your skin while saving money by not buying those imitation butters, which are much more costly than the oil or juice they are made from and offer no additional benefits.

Chapter 10 What You Need to Learn about Organic Essential Oils

What do you need to learn about organic essential oils? Organic essential oils are important Ingredients: to body butter. A particular essential oil will make the difference on whether or not it will work on your skin. Without the basic knowledge about which essential oil to choose, you might make it worse instead of better for your skin. The following are tips to avoid in choosing which essential oil to use, in the proper usage of these essential oils, and in avoiding essential oils altogether depending on circumstances.

Organic Essential Oils

Organic essential oils are generally superior to non-organic oils.

Organic oils are extracted or distilled from plants that are grown without pesticides. The therapeutic benefit and aroma of organic oils is said to be superior to oils that are non-organic

The choice is yours. You should expect to pay more for oils distilled from organic plants since it costs the provider a lot more to grow organic crops and to means maintain their land.

Make sure that your supplies are properly cleaned. Opt for glass bowls or metal bowls as they are the most sanitary. Choose to store your body butter in glass jars.

If you want to avoid your products becoming grainy later on leave your butters on the heat for 20 minutes to process it.

When melting your solid oils, if you don't have a double boiler, take a Pyrex 2-Cup Measuring Cup and set it inside a pot that is filled halfway with water.

When choosing scents for your body butter, don't be afraid to experiment. Some great options include rosemary, sweet orange, lavender, lemon and peppermint.

Don't store your product in plastic as it breaks down and can carry toxic Ingredients: into your body butter and then onto your skin. Glass is your best option.

Vitamin E won't necessarily extend the shelf life, but it will maximize the potential shelf life because it stops premature oxidization from occurring.

If you're pregnant, you should not use essential oils.

Crystallization occurs in vegetable butters sometimes forming tiny crystals when you heat and re-melt it. This can happen during the packaging process before you ever get it, or it can happen while you are working with it. Once the crystals form, the texture of the butter can become gritty. While these crystals are harmless and will melt when they come in contact with your skin, they can detract from the appearance of your body butter. To eliminate crystals, butters need to be tempered. A good body butter melts when it contacts your warm skin, so you can imagine what will happen if it is exposed to the warmth of the day. That's why whipped body butters don't travel well. Even in your home, whipped body butters might have difficulty setting or remaining fluffy during hot days.

Choose to use organic Ingredients: if you want the purest possible body butter. Some of the best prices for organic Ingredients: can be found online.

Conclusion

Congratulations! You have learned the essential list of ingredients and equipment you require to create these safe body butters. You've understood the dynamics of some of the most important essential oils, and what they can do to boost your overall health.

Most importantly, you've inherited nearly twenty body butter recipes--each with assigned benefits for particular ailments, each with beautiful fragrance and natural

Ingredients:.

You're taking charge of your own, natural way of living. Your skin will begin its youthful trek to a better future; your body will begin to fuel itself with relief after that steady stream of chemicals and irritants has halted. Here is my personal experience to inspire and guide you on your journey. My all-natural journey began a few years ago. I was tired and stressed all the time. I found myself continually turning to whatever beauty product regime was best advertised: the one that exclaimed it would help my skin look less aged and more youthful, the one that spouted that my skin would look vibrant AND my brain would be less-stressed, less frazzled--But nothing seemed to work. Around this time, I had begun to look into the Paleo diet. (Perhaps you've heard of it?) The Paleo diet creates a more natural world—one in which you turn back to what our ancestors ate for nourishment some ten thousand years ago. My body started to feel relief; I started to lose weight; and my brain started to calm with the ready intake of these healthful, good foods. And that's when I started thinking: why couldn't my beauty regime look to natural elements from the earth, as well, for nourishment and relief? I read the label on my store-bought body butter—the current one at-the-time that spouted complete and utter relief from whatever was ailing me. The Ingredients:' list was—in a word—scary. It looked sort of like the back of the sugary snacks I was tossing out of my cabinet on the road to Paleo living. If I wanted to know exactly what I was eating and putting into my body, wouldn't I want to know exactly what I was smearing over my skin—the largest organ of my body, the organ that sucked all nutrients, all chemicals, everything into my body from the rest of the world? Sure, I did. So, I started messing around, learning about essential oils. I made a lot of bad body butter recipes; I made a lot of good ones. The ones I've brought together here bring the essence of stress relief, of comfort, and of beauty. Just because you aren't spending an arm and a leg at the beauty store anymore doesn't mean you can't feel truly beautiful, truly natural. You can feel like the best version of yourself—at the height of your youth and your health. Trust me: if I can do it—I, who used to leave Bath & Body Works with 18 lotions, just to see which would work—you can do this, too. All you need is a few Ingredients—which I've outlined clearly for you—and a few drops of essential oils.

Take the wheel on your natural, clean, and vibrant lifestyle. You won't turn back. Just like I did, you'll experience:

- The youthful qualities of fresher, vibrant skin that bounces back—even after years of toxin and sun damage.

- The fresh, natural-smelling relief of some of the most wonderful essential oils. I've outlined all the benefits of my most-favorite essential oils.

- The sheer quality of each of these $5-or-less body butters. Note that you'll have to pay a bit up front, of course; but when you have a supply of butters, oils, and essential oils—all of which can be utilized for cooking and simplistic healing, as well—you can make body butters in just about an hour or less, whenever you like!

- The healing powers of each of these body butters can work to de-stress you, take away your wrinkles, and rev you with a renewed sense of vitality.

- The beauty of becoming your own woman—a woman that can create beautiful, fresh-smelling body butters at home, without the assistance of any great company. You're turning back to the earth for a renewed sense of strength and grandeur.

We have outlined the essential reasons you MUST go natural and organic to fuel yourself with good health. It allows you to look at the back of your store-bought body butters and beauty supplies for the first time and understand the intricacies of each long list of Ingredients:. What are those Ingredients: doing to your insides? You can be certain they aren't doing anything glamorous to your skin on a cellular level. You must turn them away and attempt to live a better, more natural life. You are your own woman--a woman of the natural world. Congratulations on beginning your journey. And good luck to you.

BODY SCRUBS

EASY AND NATURAL DIY RECIPES TO MAKE HOMEMADE BODY SCRUBS FOR SMOOTH, SOFT AND YOUTHFUL SKIN

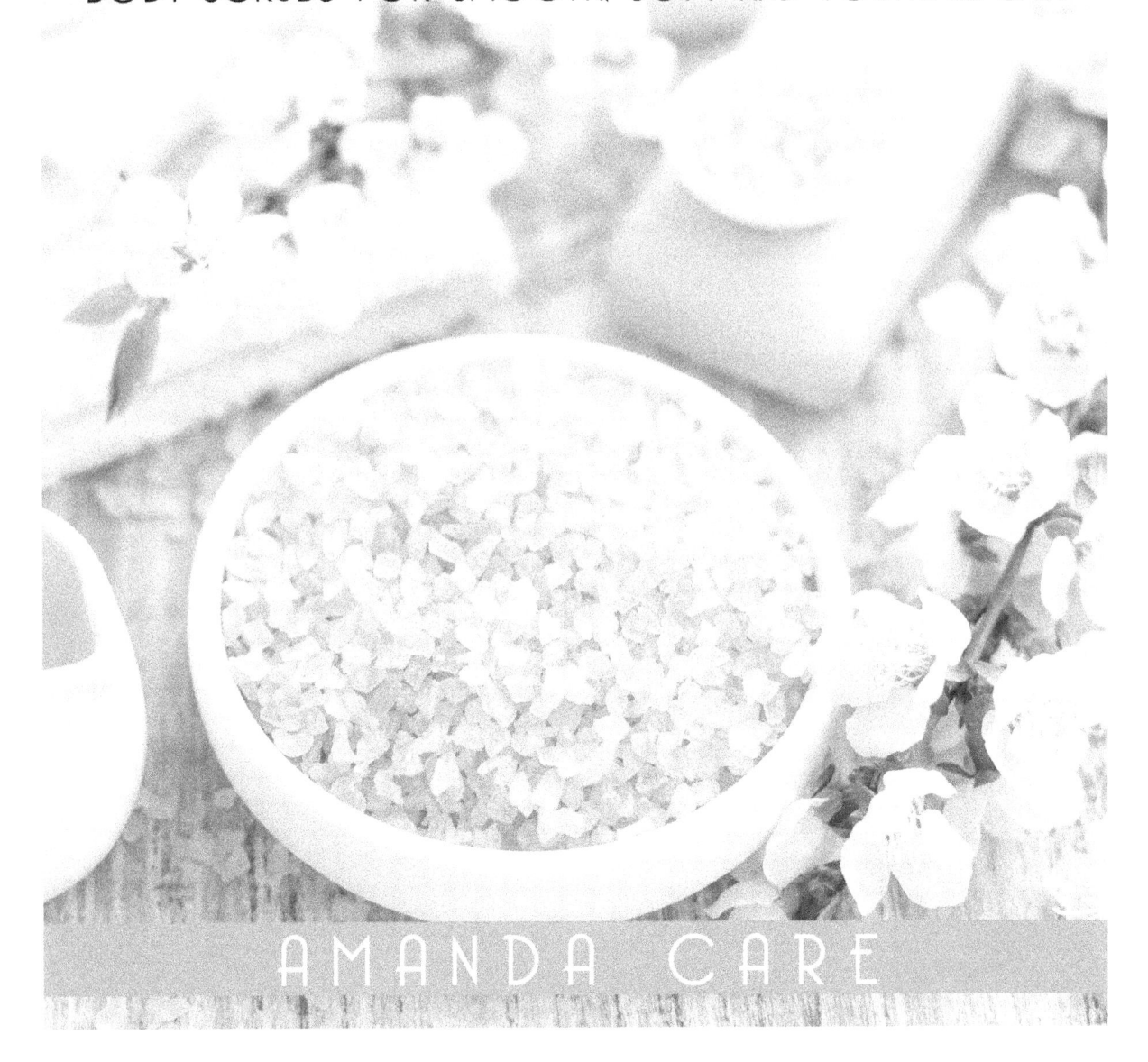

AMANDA CARE

BODY SCRUB RECIPES

Easy and natural DIY recipes to make homemade body scrubs for smooth, soft and youthful skin

Amanda Care

TABLE OF CONTENTS

INTRODUCTION **128**

CHAPTER 1 WHY USE BODY SCRUBS? **136**

CHAPTER 2 THE MAGIC OF OILS FOR SKIN CARE **146**

CHAPTER 3 INGREDIENTS AND TOOLS THAT YOU NEED TO MAKE HOMEMADE BODY SCRUBS **154**

CHAPTER 4 METHODS OF MAKING ORGANIC ESSENTIAL OILS FOR BODY SCRUBS **162**

CHAPTER 5 BASIC BODY SCRUB RECIPES **168**

CHAPTER 6 COFFEE-BASED AND FOR OILY SKIN BODY SCRUBS **178**

CHAPTER 7 OATMEAL-BASED BODY SCRUB RECIPES **188**

CHAPTER 8 SALT AND SUGAR-FREE BODY SCRUBS **196**

CHAPTER 9 FRUIT AND COFFEE-BASED SCRUB RECIPES **202**

CHAPTER 10 ADDITIONAL BODY SCRUB RECIPES **210**

CHAPTER 11 CLEANSING, NOURISHING AND HYDRATING EXFOLIANTS ... **222**

CONCLUSION **228**

Introduction

What Are Natural Body Scrubs?

Homemade natural body scrubs are simply body conditioners made up of three to four of the most wholesome ingredients. These scrubs help to exfoliate, moisturize and soften your skin and with prolonged use can totally transform the complexion, tone and overall feel of your skin.

If you have dry or damaged skin, they can help to relieve the irritation that you feel, particularly in hot or cold weather conditions. Natural body scrubs are an alternative to using ready made scrubs that you buy in the store that are often full of hidden and harmful ingredients.

My body scrubs are super easy to make and I always say to people who ask, making body scrubs is a bit like making a salad, you toss a bunch of ingredients in a bowl, throw some oil on them, give them a stir and that's it, you have your very own body scrub that will works wonders on your skin.

What's great about these scrubs is that you can create a spa like experience right in the comfort of your home and you will only pay pennies compared to what you would pay if you booked into one of those fancy spas.

There are all types of homemade body scrubs that you can make, you can make them to treat particular skin conditions or simply make them in order to completely immerse yourself in luxury ingredients that are served to do nothing else but pamper you.

These scrubs are far more beneficial to your skin than almost anything you can buy off a shelf because they are made from 100% natural ingredients, no preservatives, no additives, no harsh chemicals, zilch, nada, nothing.

I like to use things that I have in the kitchen already and often make new body scrubs right off the bat as soon as the idea enters my head. The best thing about making my own products is that I know exactly what is in them which is invaluable to me.

Now that I know about these wonderful homemade luxury scrubs, I simply cannot go back to using the store-bought products that I used to put on my skin. I can neither subject my family members to all the rubbish that they put in those products, so we all use natural homemade products in our house.

Please read about some of the hazardous and harmful chemicals that are secretly hidden in some of those store-bought products.

I haven't purchased a store-bought soap, scrub, body wash or any bathroom beauty product for the last five years. Since I started to make my own homemade body scrubs I haven't looked back and I have managed to save myself a small fortune at the same time. By the time you finish reading, you will hopefully not be in a hurry to want to buy any more of them either.

Hazardous Ingredients I Found In Store Bought Body Scrubs

Five years ago, I was motivated to start experimenting with and making my own homemade beauty products after finding out about all the harsh chemicals and toxins that are hidden in them. I learned that these toxins seep into your system through your skin and can have devastating effects on your health.

Did you know for example that some manufactures use the following toxic and harmful chemicals in their products:

- Synthetic (un-natural) fragrances
- Methlyparaben
- Oxybenzone
- Stearalkonium Chloride
- Diethanolamine
- Propylene Glycol
- Artificial colors

There are absolutely tons and tons of other harmful and toxic chemicals that they use too. I have only listed the few that I can remember. Look them up and compare them with the ingredients on your own products (if you have any store-bought products) and I think you will be surprised!

I can barely even pronounce any of the toxins and I wonder why? When I found out what was going on that was it for me, I decided to make my own products, so I knew what I was putting ON my body and IN my system.

I cannot stress enough the importance of knowing what you are putting on your skin. Make it a priority to examine the products that you currently use and cut out the ones that have these harsh chemicals in them.

List of Common Ingredients I Use & Their Health Benefits

Before I move onto the individual recipes, I would like to mention a few things first. In my true experimental nature, I don't like to be too rigid and like to create my natural products in an organic way with the ingredients I have available at the time. I am imagining you are the same and would therefore like to say that you can adapt any of the recipes to suit your individual taste and budget.

Body Scrub - How much does each recipe make?

Most of the recipes will give you enough for two applications. Some of the scrubs are for one. This is because I sometimes only like to make a quick scrub for the moment and therefore don't require as much in the way of salt, sugar, oil etc. Where this is the case you will see that I only use 1/2 cup measurements.

If you want to make more or less body scrub or you want a more solid or runny consistency for your body scrub then just experiment, adding more salt, sugar or oil to your recipe until you get the consistency that you like. It really is super easy.

I want to briefly discuss some of the basic ingredients that I use and the health benefits for each and also give you some alternative options if you don't have the same ingredients to hand.

Salt (Used as an exfoliator)

I use sea salt or dead sea salt in most of my salt body scrub recipes. You don't have to stick to the salt I use though if you don't have any of that salt at hand. You can substitute the salt I use with the salt of your choice. Other salts you can use include:

- Table Salt
- Kosher Salt (bigger salt granules)
- Epsom Salt
- Sugar (Used as an exfoliator)

- In my sweet homemade body scrub recipes nine times out of ten I use just natural organic brown sugar. Again, you are not restricted to using this (or even using organic products) and can try any type of sugar like:
- Turbinado (raw) sugar
- White sugar
- Regular brown store bought sugar
- Oil

You need a carrier oil to help bind the ingredients together and make the scrub easier to handle and spread over your body. Different oils have different skin benefits and you don't need to stick to one oil either. You can mix two oils in one scrub. If I use an oil that you don't have, you can replace it with any of the following:

- Almond Oil - Dry skin fighter full of E, A & D vitamins. Good for moisturizing and fighting the appearance of wrinkles.
- Avocado Oil - Fantastic skin boosting oil that is great for treating eczema and dry skin conditions helping to accelerate healing.
- Coconut Oil - Perfect moisturizing oil and one of the best skin softeners
- Grapeseed Oil - Good for oily and acne skin problems with known anti-aging properties
- Jojoba Oil - Good for oily skin types as it helps regulate oil production. It is a great moisturizer too and really good for stretch marks
- Olive Oil - Fantastic oil with anti-inflammatory properties. soothing and packed with skin enhancers and protectors.
- Vitamin E Oil - Great moisturizing and healing oil, good for treating scars and dark spots

Essential Oils

I use a variety of essential oils in the recipes. You can stick with mine or use your favorites, it's your body scrub and it is entirely up to you. Some of the common essential oils I use are:

- Lavender oil - Wonderful oil and one of the most common. Great for both dry and oily skin and great for creating calming scrubs. Also, very good for treating acne, wrinkles and tightening the skin.
- Tea tree oil - Natural anti-bacterial and anti-fungal oil, perfect for troublesome skin, acne, dermatitis and a range of other skin conditions.
- Chamomile - Calming and soothing oil with so many benefits. It is anti-bacterial, anti-fungal, is used as an anti-depressant and is great for making nighttime scrubs
- Geranium - This is a great stress relieving oil; it helps to relieve tension in your muscles and revive you. It is said that Geranium helps to balance you spiritually.
- Rose - Known for the effective treatment in toning and lifting the skin and fighting feelings of anxiety, thus putting you in a more relaxed state. It is also good for acne and dry skin conditions
- Lemon - Perfect for cleansing and cleaning the toxins found in your skin. It has anti-inflammatory properties as well so it can be used in a variety of scrubs. It is also totally refreshing, and you definitely feel lifted with this oil.
- Neroli - Another anxiety and stress busting oil, it is great for the nighttime with its calming effects due to its high levels of natural sedatives.

- Peppermint - For oily skin types, this oil is also great if you are feeling a bit heavy (not in weight but in how you feel!). Great for treating itchiness and muscle pains as well.

Other Ingredients I use

- Yogurt - I use it to help remove dead skin cells on my body, it moisturizes and brightens the skin.
- Oatmeal - Great skin cleanser and restorer. Good for itchy and dry skin as it helps to lock in moisture.
- Nuts - Good for tired and problematic skin. Helps to bring back natural glow.
- Honey – It has been used for thousands of years to nourish the skin, honey helps to open up and unclog the pores on your skin..
- Aloe Vera Gel - Very calming, healing gel, good for treating dry skin conditions
- Herbs - The power of natural herbs are well known. I use fresh herbs in some of my recipes because of the wonderful powers each one has.
- Fruit - Same thing, the healing benefits of fruit on the skin are well documented. I love using fresh strawberries, lime, orange, apple, banana, anything really, as long as it's fresh.

Adding color to your scrubs

Personally, I don't like to add any color to my scrubs and prefer them in their natural form however, you can add color if you wish. Some people like to add food coloring to give their scrub a richer color. Experiment and see what you prefer, remember it's up to you.

Storage of your natural body scrubs

Don't forget that we are not using any nasty preservatives in these recipes so that the scrubs won't last more than a couple of weeks in my opinion. This is when stored in the bathroom. Storing it in the fridge will prolong the life of the scrub but it will also make the scrub hard and it takes too much time to soften it and use it to bother. It's quicker for me just to make them as I need them.

When you have made your products, store them in airtight containers or glass bottles for best results.

Chapter 11 Why Use Body Scrubs?

Body scrubs are a popular skin care product used to exfoliate the skin to remove dead skin cells. It also cleanses your skin and helps to improve blood circulation throughout your body. You may hear these referred to as body exfoliants, body polish or even body gloss. A good body scrub is abrasive enough to remove the dead skin cells, but not so abrasive that it damages healthy skin.

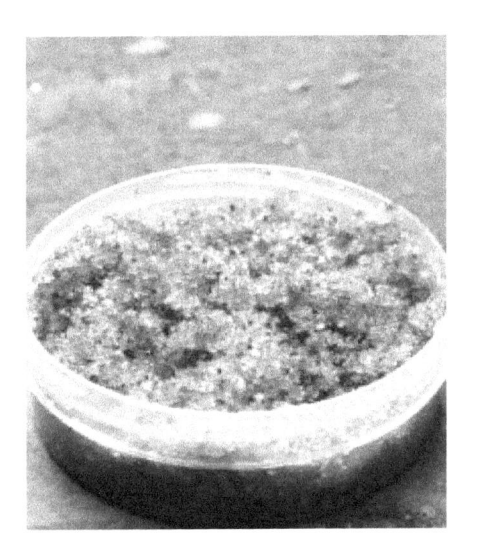

There are many benefits to body scrubs, and they have become a key ingredient to good looking, healthy skin. The removal of dead skin cells and cleansing of the skin makes you feel more refreshed and gives your skin a rejuvenated appearance. Regularly users of body scrubs report that their skin is shiny and looks much more youthful.

The average human sheds anywhere from 11,000 to 23,000 skin cells every hour. It takes between 27 and 30 days for the new skin cells to get to the top layer of your skin. These new skin cells are the youthful, fresh looking ones that make your skin look like its glowing.

With a body scrub, you slough off the old skin cells, leaving the new cells more visible. However, body scrubs can be used too much which damages the skin, so most people will use a scrub two, or maybe three, times a week to avoid damaging their skin.

One of the significant benefits of a body scrub is that it typically contains oil which acts as a moisturizer for your skin. After your body scrub, use a good quality moisturizer, and your skin will absorb it much more comfortable.

Of course, the benefits are not just limited to smoother, younger looking skin. Body scrubs also benefit your skin in many other ways, including:

Reducing the frequency of skin breakouts

Helping to reduce the appearance of age or dark spots

Reducing the appearance of large pores

Smoothing your elbows and knees

Makes hair removal much easier

Helps to prevent ingrown hairs

Smooths out razor bumps

For anyone who uses self-tanning products or has a spray tan, exfoliating with a gentle body scrub removes dead skin and prevents that blotchy look that many people end up with. These blotches, usually found on areas such as the knees and elbows, are caused by an accumulation of dead skin cells.

Although you can buy body scrubs in stores, many of these are not as good for you as you may think. A lot of these contain ingredients that are also harmful to the environment. A lot of commercially available body scrubs contain potentially harmful chemicals or even tiny plastic beads, which are the exfoliating agent. These micro-beads are under a lot of scrutiny and are now being banned in countries across the world because of the harm they do to the oceans and environment.

More and more people are moving towards natural products that are not only good for them but also good for the environment. Body scrubs are usually used in the shower, so they wash off you, going down the drain and into the world at large. Making your own body scrubs means you can use natural or even organic ingredients which are not detrimental to the environment. You can be conscious of where the products you use are sourced and the impact they have on the world around you.

Perhaps the most significant benefit of home-made body scrubs is that you have complete control over the ingredients. You can create scrubs that suit your skin type and any allergies that you may have. If you have any skin conditions, then these scrubs can be made with ingredients that alleviate those conditions. You can even make small quantities of body scrub which can give your skin what it requires on the day you use it. This control over the ingredients is terrific as you can use the right ingredients for what your skin needs, and body scrubs are neither complex or time consuming to make!

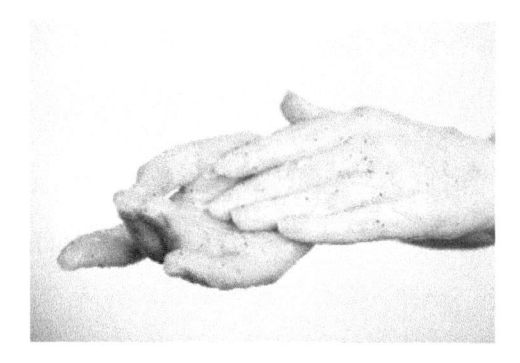

If you do have sensitive skin, then scrubs containing crushed nuts or salt are best avoided because they can cause tiny, microscopic tears in your skin. These tears can become a breeding ground for bacteria, causing acne and other skin problems.

The gentlest body scrub is made from sugar, which is not too abrasive on your skin. This is a popular scrub because it helps to reverse the early signs of aging by evening out your skin tone while removing dead skin. As you gently massage it into your skin, it improves blood circulation which increases the production of collagen and the regeneration of skin cells. This helps to prevent wrinkles and reduces other signs of aging. For anyone with susceptible skin, then an oatmeal-based scrub is best as it is incredibly gentle and kind for a wide variety of skin complaints.

Sugar scrubs are great at removing excess oil and dirt from your pores, which helps to prevent skin blemishes, acne and blackheads. By exfoliating your skin, you remove the things that spot causing bacteria feed on. Sugar scrubs can also be very helpful to reduce the symptoms of skin problems such as psoriasis and eczema.

Body scrubs should be a part of your regular beauty routine. They have a lot of benefits for your skin and can help give it a youthful shine. Using a body scrub two or three times a week will help remove dead skin cells, prevent breakouts and reduce stress. You are going to learn all about how to make your body scrubs at home, including many recipes with different base exfoliating ingredients and more. You will learn what the different ingredients used in body scrubs are, how they affect the result and how to create your body scrub recipes that are perfect for your skin.

The Exfoliant -What It Is & Why You Need It

The main ingredient in a body scrub is the exfoliant. This provides the scrub part of the product which removes the dead skin cells. Different exfoliants provide different levels of scrub. Some are more abrasive than others, and so remove more layers of skin, whereas others are much gentler. The abrasive scrubs should be used less frequently to avoid causing any damage to your skin.

The exfoliating ingredient can be anything from crushed nuts to crushed pumice stone or even coffee. However, salt and sugar are the most popular agents. You must choose one that is good for your skin and will not damage it.

Now let's talk about the different types of exfoliating agent, so you understand the differences between them.

Sugar Based Body Scrubs

This is by far the most popular exfoliating agent in body scrubs and can be anything from granulated (white) sugar to brown sugar, palm sugar or any other type of sugar. Whichever type of sugar it is, this provides a gentler scrub which can be used more frequently than harsher scrubs, hence its popularity. Sugar based scrubs have an oil or glycerin product added which turns it into a paste that can then be used on your skin.

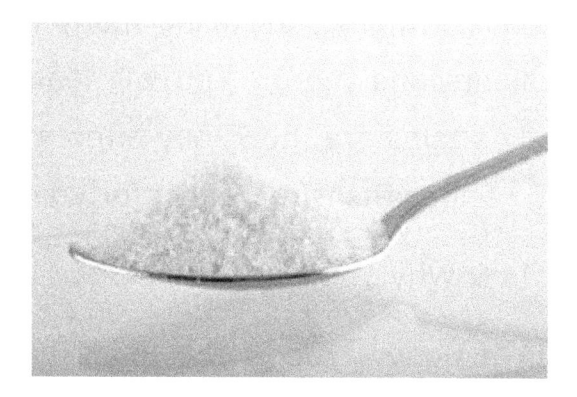

The sugar granule is round, which means it cannot cut the skin as salt granules can. Sugar based scrubs are therefore much gentler, and the best choice for sensitive skin and are the only option for facial scrubs. Sugar also dissolves easily in hot water, which also helps them to be less abrasive.

Although sugar scrubs do not provide the mineral benefits of salt scrubs, they are less drying to the skin. If you can use less refined versions of sugar, then you can get some nutrient benefits from it.

Sugar also contains glycolic acid which helps to protect your skin from harmful toxins, making it important in your regular beauty routine. Sugar can come in different grain sizes from fine to medium to coarse, which will have a different effect on your skin.

Body scrubs based on sugar are the most popular type of scrub because they are gentle and good for your skin. Many people prefer sugar-based scrubs because they are less abrasive and are ideal for anyone with sensitive skin.

Salt Based Scrubs

Body scrubs using salt as the exfoliating agent are much more abrasive than sugar-based scrubs and so are used less frequently. These scrubs are more rejuvenating and will bring toxins to the surface of the skin. Depending on your requirements, you can use different grades of sea salt to give different levels of abrasiveness.

Salt crystals are not round in shape, instead having sharp edges which gives them their abrasive nature. Unlike sugar-based scrubs, salts offer therapeutic and mineralization benefits. The most commonly used salt is sea salt, which is a natural purifier that works to remove toxins that block your pores.

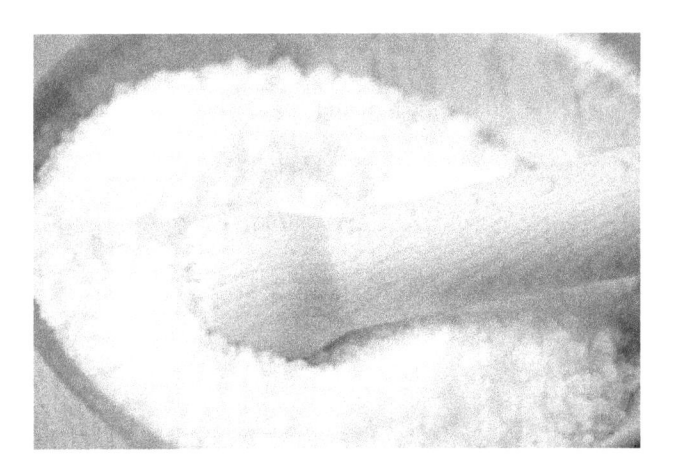

This helps your skin to breath better, tightens it, promotes better circulation and improves its texture.

Coarser salts provide a more abrasive scrub and are great to use on areas such as your feet and elbows. They are very good for occasional use to soften dry or calloused skin or to detoxify your skin. Because they are much more abrasive, salt-based scrubs tend to be used less frequently, usually only once a week to avoid causing any damage. After a salt scrub, apply a good quality moisturizer in the form of a body butter, cream or oil. If you have irritated or damaged skin, it is best to avoid salt scrubs completely as they sting!

There are many different types of salt, but there are five main salts used in beauty products. Sea salt is the most popular salt and is made by dehydrating seawater and collecting the salt that is left behind. The five main sea salts are:

1)   Dead Sea Salt – This comes from the Dead Sea which is located in the Middle East, between Israel and Jordan. This salt is known to for its therapeutic effects, and people travel thousands of miles to swim in the Dead Sea and benefit from its healing properties.

2)   Natural Black Salt – This is formed when lava reaches seawater and is harvested from cooled lava flows. Most black salt comes from Hawaii, and it is very high in minerals and antioxidants. It contains a lot of sulfur, which is reflected in the mild odor it gives off and has a coarse texture, so is an ideal exfoliant.

3)   Pink Himalayan Salt – Although technically not sea salt, this is a much sought after salt which has recently become popular in cooking. It is found, as you can guess, in the Himalaya mountains and is very rich in halite and iron. It is very popular in skin care products because of its mineral content.

4)   Maldonado Salt – This salt originates from the United Kingdom. It is made from dehydrating saltwater to produce pyramid-shaped salt

crystals. This salt is pure white and is popular in both cooking and beauty therapy.

5) Epsom Salt – While technically not a salt, it is extremely popular in beauty products and works very well in body scrubs. Epsom salt is made up of magnesium sulfate and is well known as a relaxing bath salt. It plumps up your skin, leaving it feeling smooth and supple.

Chapter 12 The Magic of Oils for Skin Care

If you have odious skin nothing is more important than good natural skin care. While dry skin needs extreme humidity, those with oily skin suffer from excessive moisture like oil and the problems involved. The good news is that normal, oily skin care will solve these problems.

The lack of signs of aging as well as dry skin is one of the commonly overlooked benefits of fatty skin. This is because the oil drums have extra moisture. Treatment for fat skin combines the anti-aging benefits of fatty skin with the removal of excess moisture. Fat skin treatment will also make your skin beautiful.

Oily skin patients also need washing of their faces and are typically prone to acne. Overactive oil glands can lead to acne if proper care for the oily skin is not taken. Grime and debris collect quickly on oily skin and block pores, which promote bacterial growth and acne development.

Through washing your skin oily you can help prevent acne through removing excess oil. Cleanse the skin of carbon and warm water ingredients for the best results. A natural cleanser removes dirt and grime and performs miracles on oily skin.

Upon washing, clean your face with warm water and then apply a toner or an astringent made from a natural ingredient recipe. Excess oil can be absorbed by natural toner without changing the pH of your skin or losing your essential moisture face.

Natural oily skin care with natural ingredients is much safer than using tough, skin irritating substances. Chemical products for skin care can often lead to a severe oily skin condition called Seborrhea.

For lack of skin moisture, seborrhea produces oil under the skin surface through the use of artificial skin care products that are dry. The top layer dries due to the oxidation of the chemical skin care product.

This prevents oil from flowing from oil glands, blocking pores and causing acne. Natural oily treatment of skin made from natural ingredients is good for oily skin and helps prevent Seborrhea infection.

To people with oily skin who are also scaly, an oily skin scrub made from natural ingredients should be used. A natural scrub exfoliates your skin by removing essential moisture.

Another great option for oily skin care is a natural facial mask. Excess oil is covered gently with natural clay masks. Apply a natural mask with the natural ingredients of a recipe, and rinse with warm water. A moisturizer is then applied with natural oily skin treatment.

Experiment with natural skin care by making your oily skin care products home with recipes and natural ingredients. Through playing with various recipes, you can find the natural ingredients that work best for your fat skin. The more ingredients and recipes you are using, the better the natural oily skin treatment.

One of the main differences among classical skin care and natural or organic skin care is that they are not "solid" ingredients, such as green tea or vitamin c, that account for up to 5% of products, but the fundamental ingredients.

For natural skin care, the essential ingredients are often a mixture of vegetable oil with butter or wax, rather than traditional skin care synthetic ingredients. The use of essential oils greatly helps the skin.

Fundamental oils contain nutrients including vitamins, minerals and essential fats, which help and cultivate the skin rather than be an inert synthetic carrier for the active ingredients. I would go to mention essential oils as active ingredients in skin care.

Furthermore, up to 95% of all-natural ingredients have a protective "aging" effect on the skin. In comparison, the synthetic basic ingredients in modern skin care have no major therapeutic benefit.

Many factors affect the absorption of topical ingredients into the skin and, besides, many topical creams only lie on the surface of the skin, effectively plumping skin cells into their surface.

The skin is highly absorbent and relatively permeable to fats soluble and water-soluble. Fat soluble ingredients like oils are absorbed more quickly to feed the skin and have better effect on the cell membrane and the skin matrices.

Instead of having a' top' effect, oil can also hold essential oils, phytonutrients, vitamins and minerals in the skin as carriers. Oils also help to avoid skin dehydration by providing an effective barrier to water loss, leading to more hydrated plumber.

That carrier oil is absorbed by viscosity or thickness with thicker oils which tend to penetrate the skin slowly. Fine light oils can be used on the face in general as they absorb quickly and easily penetrate the skin without feeling grateful. Heavier oils are ideal for dry skin, skin on the body, like bath oils and massage oils.

The degree of unsaturation also influences oil absorption. The polyunsaturated fat the higher the absorption the oil produces. The Rose hip oil is high in polyunsaturated fats. It has a fairly low viscosity, suitable for use in the face serum or cream, because it absorbs easily into the skin.

Cold-pressed oils are more unsaturated than heat-extracted oils and are therefore preferable. Cold pressing involves putting the noodle or seed into an "expeller" that dries out the oil.

Any heat generated by friction does not harm the oil or its components. Heat extraction requires up to 200 ° C temperatures, which dramatically increases oil yield, which makes it much more profitable but also destroys oil nutrients. High temperatures destroy unsaturated fatty acids easily and therefore heat extracted oil levels are significantly lower. While these oils are widely used in cooking oils, the medicinal effects of the cold-pressed variety should be avoided for use in the skin and aromatherapy.

A common misconception is that adding oils on the skin only worsens oily skin and creates more congestion. Heavier oils may be placed on the skin surface longer before absorption, which is not suitable for oily skin. Nevertheless, the smaller, less viscous oils are consumed very easily and often do not contribute to the balance of oil for the skin.

Instead of being on the surface layer, the oils are easily absorbed into the skin. They are unlikely to cause or exacerbate irritation. However, waxes and butter are the basis of many natural skin care products.

Although they are extremely beneficial to the skin, they are more likely to be on the surface. They are therefore more likely to contribute if there is already a problem of pollution. These are unlikely to cause irritation that has not existed in the past and the skin response depends on the type of skin. The ratio of waxes to butter to oils in different skin types varies. If you are unsure of which substance to use for your skin type, the manufacturer or supplier will be most suitable for your skin type.

There are great deals of healthy carrier oils used both in skin moisturizers and serums and the variety of natural products available which are that with nutritious base oils. Various oils are appropriate for various types of skin, so knowing some basic facts about base oils allows you to find the best drug for your skin.

Sweet Almond Oil

-A common skin care oil that is rich in nutrients such as vitamin E, unsaturated fats and essential fatty acids. It has a softening effect on the skin and is good for massage lubrication because it is not absorbed quickly while it is not heavy oil.

Olive Oil

-A heavier oil rich in oleic acid and monounsaturated fats. Extra virgin olive oil originates from the first pressing of olives. It is colored in dark green suggesting the existence of polyphenol antioxidants.

It is suitable for use with dry skin because it helps to balance the cell membrane to improve skin moisture retention. Squalene, a moisturizing and anti-inflammatory agent, also contains olive oil ideally suited for skin conditions such as psoriasis and eczema.

Tamanu Oil

-Tamanu Oil has powerful healing properties in its unique ability to promote new skin tissue development. Oil historically used for skin and mucous membranes by the Polynesians may sustain cuts, burns, skin cracks, slices, dry skin, and wounds.

Tamanu is used for beauty procedures, moderate antibiotics and anti-inflammatory behaviors 2. It is therefore used in defensive as well as regenerative products for restoring the appearance of the skin.

Primrose Evening Oil

-Primrose Evening Oil (EPO) is a precious source of gamma linoleic acid, an essential fatty acid with a strong anti-inflammatory effect. Useful for dry, impaired, sensitive skin EPO helps maintain healthy functions of the skin barrier. It is also topically useful for psoriasis and eczema.

Rosehip Oil

-Rosehip oil is wonderful with up to 80% essential fatty acid content and is absorbed very quickly by the skin. Rosehip encourages skin regeneration and repair and is known for its skin benefits, particularly in the treatment of scars and burns. It is also renowned for its rehydration and the treatment of dry, aged and wrinkled skin.

Jojoba Oil

-Rather than an oil, Jojoba oil is skinny and easily absorbed into the skin. It is light and non-greasy and is ideal for serums and creams. Jojoba resembles skin sebum closely and is therefore helpful to skin and scalp disorders, including psoriasis and eczema. It is moisturizing, soothing and ideal for all skin types with outstanding emollient properties.

Cocoon Oil

–One of the most robust and most durable oils, cocoon is suitable for the application of hair and body. It is suitable for dry and rough skin with moisturizing and softening properties. Coconut oil also has cooling properties and is therefore useful for goods after sun treatment 1.

Avocado Oil

-Intense in color and dour, avocado oil is not appropriate for everybody in the skin. It is rich in lecithin, vitamin D, E and A however in its unrefined form. It offers useful sun protection and skin nutrition. Avocado oil is suitable for drying skins.

Sea Buckthorn Oil

-Bright color orange, Sea Buckthorn Oil is high in beta carotene, with Rose Hip only in vitamin C. It is also very high in fatty acids. A vibrant mix of nutrients ensures that the base oil in your skin is extremely beneficial. It's easy to absorb and valid for all skin types with hydrating, anti-inflammatory and restore properties.

Chapter 13 Ingredients and Tools That You Need To Make Homemade Body Scrubs

There are necessarily three main ingredients that are required for a successful body scrub: exfoliant, carrier oil and essential oil. There are many options within these three categories to choose from. Therefore, it's not uncommon for those new to the whole homemade body scrub scene to feel a bit intimidated by all the choices. Thankfully, the following information will help get you acquainted with the basic ingredients of body scrubs, so you're not going into the process blind.

1. Exfoliant

While sugar and salt are the two most common ingredients used as an exfoliant in homemade scrubs, there is actually various other ingredients that work well as an exfoliant. Ground coffee and oatmeal are two popular alternatives to sugar and salt.

Ground coffee not only gives the body scrub a pleasant aroma, but also provides benefits to the skin. Furthermore, the caffeine naturally found in coffee is a vasoconstrictor. In layman's terms, caffeine causes the blood vessels to constrict, which helps to reduce – albeit temporarily – rosacea and varicose veins.

Oatmeal is an extremely gentle exfoliant. In fact, it is the gentlest exfoliant for body scrubs. Oatmeal is also an emollient, which means it hydrates and softens the skin. For decades, people have used oatmeal as a home remedy for itchy, dry skin. Unlike the other exfoliants, water can be used as a carrier oil for oatmeal body scrubs.

Flax meal, almond meal, ground nutshells, buckwheat, wheat bran, cornmeal and rice bran also work well as an exfoliant for your homemade body scrubs.

2. Carrier Oil

Carrier oil – sometimes called base oil – is essentially what holds the ingredients of the body scrub together while acting as a moisturizer for the skin. As with exfoliants, there are a wide array of carrier oils to choose from, many with different benefits to consider. Most recipes – expect for those that tackle dry skin – generally call for a carrier oil that has a thin consistency, which means it washes off the skin easily and doesn't leave a greasy residue behind.

Olive Oil is probably the easiest carrier oil to get your hands on, and it's rather inexpensive to boot. If you use olive oil for your homemade body scrub, make sure to choose the lightest grade available, so the oil's natural scent doesn't cover up the smell of any essential oils you are using in the recipe. Olive oil has a shelf life of about a year.

Sunflower oil has a thin consistency, is practically odorless and can penetrate the skin. In addition, sunflower oil is typically less expensive than other carrier oils and has about a 12 month shelf life.

Grape seed oil is a very thin oil that absorbs easily and has a faint, sweet aroma. Its shelf life is typically between 6 and 12 months.

Sweet almond oil has a nutty, somewhat sweet fragrance. This medium consistency oil absorbs into the skin quickly and has a shelf life of up to 12 months.

Jojoba oil is known for its moisturizing capabilities without leaving behind a greasy residue on your skin. It works great for sensitive skin and has a stable shelf life that increases when added to other carrier oils.

Hazelnut oil is a nutty-smelling carrier oil with a thin consistency that will leave a film on your skin. Its shelf is around 12 months.

Vitamin E oil is a light, soft option for body scrubs. Unfortunately, it is rather expensive, and some DIYers choose to use a bit of this oil with another carrier oil to make it last longer.

Kukui Oil and its thin consistency absorb well into the skin. It has a sweet yet light nutty aroma and shelf life of about 12-months.

Macadamia nut oil is a thick oil that will leave an oily film behind. This nutty-smelling oil has a shelf life of 12-months and works best for dry skin.

Keep in mind that those are only some of the possible carrier oils you can use for your homemade body scrub.

3. Essential Oils

While essential oils can often be eliminated from the recipe, they do provide many benefits that make their presence invaluable to the body scrub. Essential oils – which are derived from and contain the compounds of plants – not only give the body scrub a pleasant aroma, they are also beneficial for your health.

Sugar Vs. Salt: What Is The Difference Between The Two In Your Homemade Body Scrubs?

Sugar and salt have a similar appearance and can be hard to distinguish by looks alone. When they are used in a body scrub, however, you can quickly tell the difference between the two. Both contain coarse grains that work as an all-natural exfoliator to help remove the dead cells that accumulate on the top layer of your skin. Once the dead cells are removed, your skin will appear rejuvenated, fresh and glowing. However, both sugar and salt have their own specific benefits that you should consider when choosing your ingredients.

Salt For Homemade Body Scrubs

Salt is more abrasive than its sweeter counterpart is and works best for troubled areas, such as elbows and heels. Salt also absorbs oil, which makes it ideal for skin plagued with acne. Salt naturally has anti-viral and anti-bacterial properties, and a body scrub containing salt can help improve circulation when rubbed over your skin. Since salt is more abrasive than sugar, it works better to remove the layer of dead cells on rough, dry skin. Another thing to consider is that unlike sugar scrubs, homemade scrubs made with salt are not sticky and usually fall off while rubbing into the skin. This can lead to excessive waste of the scrub.

Sugar For Homemade Body Scrubs

While sugar is still an exfoliator, it is gentler than salt. This is due to the sugar granules being round, which means it doesn't cut into the skin. Its gentle nature makes sugar the better ingredient for people with sensitive skin. Furthermore, sugar body scrub can be safely used on the face. The granules in the sugar scrubs dissolve easily in hot water, but don't contain the mineral benefits that you receive with salt scrubs. Sugar scrubs, however, are less drying and suitable for all skin conditions and types. Sugar also naturally contains glycolic acid, which helps to protect your skin from harmful toxins and is vitally important for skin health.

Glycolic acid also can moisturize and condition. Sugar scrubs are stickier and softer than salt scrubs and will remain on your skin while applying. This allows the oils to stay put longer, giving them time to work their magic.

Most basic sugar-based body scrubs only include olive oil, while others contain a few drops of essential oils. This type of body scrub is gentle enough for the skin. If you are thinking that sugar's granules are too harsh, they actually are not. For one thing, there are many types of sugars, and in making a homemade body scrub, nothing requires you to use granulated sugar. You can use white sugar, which is less grainy. Sugar scrub is not at all harsh on the skin, but it is rough enough for the right exfoliating action. The particles of brown sugar, specifically, are not big enough to cause tears in the pores while it exfoliates the skin.

Which Is The Best Ingredient To Use For Your Homemade Scrub?

It all really depends on your specific situation. Armed with the information above, you should be able to choose the right ingredient for your needs. For example, if Aunt Deloris complains about the bottom of her feet being rough, use salt in her batch and save the sugar for your family members who have sensitive skin.

Making homemade body scrubs is a no-sweat DIY activity that anybody can do. It does not require much of your time and it will definitely not get in the way of family or work. Simply mixing ingredients together makes almost all homemade body scrubs. Some recipes will require the use of liquefied oils, which is achieved by melting oil under low heat in a saucepan. Don't worry; this is not a difficult task since it will only take a few minutes. In any case, here are some of the things you need to know about making your own body scrub at home.

What Equipment Do You Need To Make Homemade Body Scrubs

The only equipment you will need for making your own body scrub is the usual measuring utensils: measuring cup, tablespoon and teaspoon. You will definitely need a small mixing bowl and a spoon or whisk, if you prefer, for combining your ingredients. Most people prefer hand mixing the ingredients while wearing gloves. Occasionally, a small saucepan, mortar and pestle, or a food processor or blender will be needed.

How To Store Your Homemade Scrub Properly

Powdered Vitamin E or Vitamin E oil is an ingredient to consider in making any kind of homemade body scrub. It will help lengthen the shelf life of your scrub. The Vitamin E will retain the moisture of the body scrub and serve as a natural preservative. When storing your homemade body scrub, make sure that the lid is tight. Also, each time you use the scrub, do not let water get into the mixture because it will give way to molds. Before cupping a handful of body scrub from the container, make sure that your hands are dry to prevent water from getting into the mixture.

The Average Shelf-Life Of Your Homemade Scrub

Most homemade body scrubs are best used within the month, since the measurement of the ingredients only yield an average of 1 to 2 cups of body scrub. Body scrubs with fresh fruit ingredients are good to use within the week. Without the effects of water, a homemade body scrub without fresh fruit ingredients can last an average of 2 to 6 months. Adding Vitamin E into the recipe and replacing the lid tightly after every use will help ensure a 6-month shelf life.

How To Apply Your Homemade Scrub Properly

Body scrub is not a daily regimen, mainly because it can cause damage to the younger skin layer exposed from the previous exfoliation. It is highly recommended to use body scrub only once or twice a week. It is not meant to be a vigorous skin treatment but more of a gentle scrubbing cream. It is meant to gently and neatly peel away the damaged and dead skin cells.

When applying body scrub to your skin, do it in a circular motion. This helps the skin absorb the nutrients evenly and prevents abrasive scrubs from tearing at sensitive or large skin pores. Rubbing back and forth in one direction causes redness and tearing of the skin. Some body scrub recipes will still cause redness no matter how gently you apply it. Do not worry when this happens since it only means that the old, damaged surface of the skin has been removed!

SKIN CARE

Chapter 14 Methods of Making Organic Essential Oils for Body Scrubs

Essential oils are one of the main components of various skin care and beauty products. They are usually derived from plants that have healing and moisturizing properties. Although it is cheaper and more convenient to purchase readily distilled and bottled essential oils from health stores, it is better to use something that is natural and has no artificial chemicals.

Learning how to make natural homemade essential oils is one key to making your own organic skin care products such as facial scrubs. It is important to have the proper knowledge in making essential oils before proceeding to the actual process. This is to ensure that you will obtain the best and safest quality of essential oil.

There are a few ways to make essential oils. One of them is the process called expression. This process involves the mechanical pressing of fruits or plant material to express the juice or the oil. Organically grown products are passed through rolling press or cold press machine to obtain the juice and oil. Further processing is needed to separate the extracted juice from the essential oil.

Another process to make essential oil is by steam distillation. One way to do this process is by putting the organic plant into a container and placing it in boiling water to acquire the oil. Another way to do steam distillation is by simply putting the pieces of organically grown product into the boiling water. The oil will separate from the water after it was extracted from the plant though boiling. Another process is through steaming. It is by putting organic plant material into a steamer and steaming it to obtain the essential oil.

There are also some important pointers to remember before making essential oils.

You have to make sure that the plant product that you will be using is really organically grown and is free from chemicals such as herbicides, fungicides, and pesticides.

You can use either dried or fresh organic plants.

You must not overheat or over dry the plant material to avoid oil loss. The more heat that is applied to the plant while drying, the more likely it is to lose its oil content. You must not dry it under direct sunlight. You can dry it in a shadier location to allow slow drying. It is also advisable to immediately distill the plant material right after drying.

The best plant materials that you can use are citrus rinds, herbs, flower petals and spices.You must harvest the plant material on the right time to ensure the quality and quantity of oils that you will obtain.

Handle the plant material with extra care because the parts in which the oils are in (veins, hairs and oil glands) are most delicate. Handle the plant material as little as possible to avoid destroying these parts.

Flower petals are recommended to be distilled right after picking and do not require drying.

The finished product of your homemade essential oil can be much milder that store-bought oil. Keep in mind to store the essential oil in a cool dark place. Put it in a dark-colored glass or stainless-steel bottle or container to preserve its quality.Homemade essential oils are ONLY recommended for use in making skin care products and are not for cooking and aromatherapy. Before applying the essential oil onto the skin, you may want to dilute it with a carrier oil such as grape seed or almond oil. This is because the essential oil is concentrated. You can dilute it during the bottling process, but dilution will decrease the shelf life of the essential oil. Carrier oils have shorter shelf life than essential oils.

Do not ingest essential oils.

Homemade essential oil that is obtained through distillation may not be effective for therapeutic use. It is because the heat used in distillation destroys the quality and therapeutic properties of the oil.

After the distillation process and collection of essential oil, you can also use the hydrosol or the water which was separated from the oil. It can be used for other purposes or you can use it for the next batch of distillation. But if you choose not to use it, you can simply discard it.

Now that we are done with the basic knowledge in making essential oil, we may now discuss the various methods of making essential oil.

Grinding and Boiling

In this process, you will need to use a linen or cotton cloth bag in which you will be putting the plant material. You also need to grind the organic plant bits before putting it into the bag. After putting it into the bag, you have to tie the bag to keep the plant pieces inside of it while boiling. Pour enough amount of distilled water in a pot before putting the bag. Bring it to a boil and then lower the heat. Let it simmer for 24 hours to allow the oil to be extracted very well. After that, you need to squeeze off the excess liquid from the bag and scoop the extracted oils from the water's surface. Pour the oil into a dark-colored glass bottle and cover it with cloth. Let it sit for about seven days to let excess water to evaporate. Then, you can place a secure lid to let it keep for until a year.

Mixing With Oil

You can also make your own natural essential oil by stirring about half an ounce of your chosen plant pieces with two cups of grape seed, almond, olive or jojoba oil. After stirring the components together, you need to cook it in a crock pot on low fire for six hours. Then, you have to strain it with cheese cloth (unbleached) before pouring it in a dark-colored glass container with an airtight lid. It will keep for up to six months.

Soaking in Alcohol

You will need to immerse the organic plant material in a capped bottle of rubbing alcohol to do this method. Let it soak for about 2 weeks. After soaking, transfer it into a container with large opening to let the alcohol evaporate. Once the alcohol is gone, you can now obtain the essential oil and pour it in a dark-colored glass bottle. This will keep for up to six months. It is very important to remember that the essential oil gathered through this process should NOT be ingested.

Boiling

In this process, you need to pour some distilled water into a crock pot before putting the organic plant pieces. Then, you have to cook it for 24 hours on low fire. After this, let the crock pot stay uncovered and set it aside for about a week. Then, gather the oil from the surface of water and transfer it into a dark-colored glass bottle. Let the excess water evaporate by covering it with a small cloth for about a week. It will keep for about a year.

Soaking in Oil

Prepare a big glass bottle and fill half of it with oil. You can use almond, grape seed, olive or jojoba oil. Choose any organic plant material and put as much as possible into the glass bottle. Cover it and store it for 24 hours in a cool, dark place. Shake and strain it with cheese cloth after 3 days. Transfer the oil into a dark-colored glass bottle. It can keep for about six months. You can strengthen its scent by adding more plant bits and repeating the process.

Soaking in Vinegar and Oil

Put half teaspoon of white vinegar, half cup of oil (almond, grape seed, olive or jojoba) and a tablespoon of plant pieces into a small bottle with cover. For about three weeks, let it sit in a warm location. Shake it vigorously twice each day. Then, strain it with cheese cloth (unbleached) before pouring into a dark-colored glass bottle. It will keep for about six months.

Chapter 15 Basic Body Scrub Recipes

Your Go-To Basic Scrub

This easy-to-recreate basic scrub includes ingredients you are likely to have in your kitchen. If you don't stock white sugar, you can substitute brown. Sugar is very beneficial when applied to the skin for a variety of reasons. One of the biggest are the alpha hydroxy acids (AHAs) that it contains. This is the good stuff that is going to reduce those wrinkles and create a nice even tone!

Makes: 18 ounces

Ingredients

1 ½ cups organic cane sugar

¾ cup extra virgin olive oil

1 teaspoon vanilla extract

Directions

Combine the ingredients in an airtight jar, mix well, and store in a cool place.

Moisten the skin and scrub with the mixture, wash off.

Green Tea Scrub

Green tea oil provides numerous benefits to the skin. It has been used for everything from treating itching to a light form of UV protection. Its amazing antioxidant qualities make it an age-defying powerhouse. This green tea scrub provides just the right amount of anti-aging oil to green tea balance.

Makes: 18 ounces

Ingredients

1 ½ cups organic cane sugar - ¾ cup coconut oil

1 tablespoon green tea essential oil - 1 teaspoon tea tree oil

Directions

Combine the ingredients in an airtight jar, mix well, and store in a cool place.

Moisten the skin and scrub with the mixture, wash off.

Chocolate Scrub

Cocoa not only smells divine, but it is also fantastic for the skin. Chocolate masks and baths have become popular due to cocoa's inherent antioxidant capabilities. When applied to the skin, these help to rid the body of skin-damaging free radicals.

Makes: 16 ounces

Ingredients

3 tablespoons organic cocoa powder - 1 teaspoon cocoa essential oil

1 ¼ cups organic cane sugar

¾ cup coconut oil

Directions

Combine the ingredients in an airtight jar, mix well, and store in a cool place.

Moisten the skin and scrub with the mixture, wash off.

Lemon Scrub

Drop a little lemon into your scrub, and you'll see it do amazing things for your skin – like magic. Rub the lemony scrub onto your elbows and knees and watch the dark spots disappear! Additionally, lemon's astringent properties help to clean the skin and make it brighter truly.

Makes: 12 ounces

Ingredients 2 teaspoons lemon peel, grated 1 tablespoon lemon juice

1 cup organic cane sugar 2 teaspoons vitamin E oil ½ cup coconut oil

Directions

Combine the ingredients in an airtight jar, mix well, and store in a cool place.

Moisten the skin and scrub with the mixture, wash off.

Mint Chocolate Scrub

Scrub this on your body in the morning and be prepared to have the wheels in your head turning at ultimate speeds all day! The scent of peppermint has a big, positive affect on mental function in ways such as improving memory and focus.

Makes: 12 ounces

Ingredients 1 cup organic cane sugar ½ cup almond oil

2 tablespoons pure cocoa powder 1 teaspoon peppermint essential oil

Directions

Combine the ingredients in an airtight jar, mix well, and store in a cool place.

Moisten the skin and scrub with the mixture, wash off.

Epsom Foot Scrub

Dry, hardened spots on the skin are terrible to touch and pretty horrible to look at. They can be disheartening personally and quite embarrassing. This is why you must absolutely use this scrub to make your feet beautiful and lovely. Epsom salt is anti-fungal and helps to deodorize feet. In addition, the minerals also help to alleviate pain and discomfort. Your feet work hard for you, so it is definitely time to show them some love.

Makes: 12 ounces

Ingredients ¾ cup Epsom salt ¼ cup sea salt ½ cup coconut oil

Directions

Combine the ingredients in an airtight jar, mix well, and store in a cool place. Moisten the skin and scrub with the mixture, wash off.

Rice And Honey Whitening Body Scrub

Rice powder has excellent exfoliating properties, and it also helps in brightening skin tone. Honey is one of the best organic applications for your skin. It works as an antibacterial and anti-aging product. It opens up the pores and it is a good natural moisturizer that soothes your skin. It makes your skin glow and makes it soft and supple to touch.

Makes: 12 ounces

Ingredients 1 cup rice, coarsely ground 3 tablespoons honey

10-12 drops almond oil (use only for dry skin)

Directions

Combine the ingredients in an airtight jar, mix well, and store in a cool place. Moisten the skin and scrub with the mixture for a couple of minutes, then wash it off.

Summer Red Lentil Body Scrub

Rose water helps you feel refreshed during summertime. It provides relief for itchiness or a burning sensation. Honey is a good moisturizer, an antioxidant, and an antibacterial too. It suits all types of skin and makes your skin supple. The red lentils help remove dead skin cells from your skin and also give to add a healthy glow.

Makes: 12 ounces

Ingredients ½ cup red lentils, coarsely ground 3 tablespoons honey

2 tablespoons rose water

Directions

Combine ingredients in an airtight jar, mix well and store in a cool place.

Moisten skin and scrub with mixture, wash off.

Red Lentil Body Scrub For Winter

Winter can rob your skin of its natural moisture. If you have dry skin, then moisturizing frequently is important. That is where organic ghee comes to the rescue – a heavy duty natural skin moisturizer. It works wonders on dry skin, making it soft and supple. The red lentils help remove dead skin cells and also give you a healthy glow.

Makes: 12 ounces

Ingredients 1 cup red lentils, coarsely ground ½ cup ghee

Rose essential oil (since ghee can have a strong aroma)

Directions

Combine the ingredients in an airtight jar, mix well, and store in a cool place.

Moisten the skin and scrub with the mixture, wash off.

Face Whitening Scrub For Dry Skin

Milk is a natural skin moisturizer, and it's great for dry skin. People with oily skin should avoid this scrub, as it will make your face oilier. Rice powder helps in getting rid of dead skin cells and is also known to whiten your skin tone. This scrub is best used at night.

Makes: 12 ounces

Ingredients

½ cup rice, coarsely powdered - ½ cup lukewarm milk

Directions

Mix the rice powder and milk together in a bowl to form a paste.

Before bed, apply it on the face and scrub in a circular motion.

Wash it off with lukewarm water. Your face may feel a bit oily for the time being, but the natural oils from the milk will be absorbed into your skin, and you will be left with a fresh and dewy face the next morning.

Lemon Lavender Body Scrub

Scrubs are not just for getting rid of dead skin cells. Body scrubs are also known to help relieve tension and help the body relax. Epsom salt, when used in a scrub, relaxes your muscles and also helps reduce inflammation. Olive oil keeps the skin moist. Lemon juice acts as a bleaching agent, while the lavender helps you relax your senses. Used all together, this relaxing body scrub is just what you need for both body and mind after a tough day.

Makes: 12 ounces

Ingredients

1 ¼ cups Epsom salt or coarse salt crystals

¼ cup olive oil

¼ cup lemon juice

10 drops lavender essential oil

Directions

Combine the ingredients in an airtight jar, mix well, and store in a cool place.

Moisten the skin and scrub with the mixture, wash off.

Anti-Inflammatory Body Scrub

Turmeric has anti-inflammatory and antibacterial properties that soothe your skin and help fight skin bacteria. Essential oils (depending on the type you choose) have their own skincare and relaxation benefits. Sugar and salt will help get rid of dead skin cells.

Makes: 25 ounces

Ingredients:

1 ½ cups salt

1 ½ cups sugar

3 tablespoons turmeric powder

6-8 drops essential oil of your choice

Directions

Combine the ingredients in an airtight jar, mix well, and store in a cool place.

Moisten the skin and scrub with the mixture, wash off.

Scrub For Sensitive Skin

Avocado is rich in natural oils that help moisturize skin. Cucumber is known for its oil removal properties and is also a natural coolant. It has skin whitening properties as well, and it gives relief to burns and other skin inflammations. Brown sugar is an excellent dead skin cell remover.

Makes: 12 ounces

Ingredients

1 medium cucumber, chopped

1 cup brown sugar

½ cup avocado oil

Directions

Blend the cucumber pieces in a blender until smooth.

In a bowl, combine the blended cucumber, avocado oil, and brown sugar. Rub the mixture gently all over your body. Leave it on for 3-4 minutes. Wash with lukewarm water.

Scrub For Soothing Sore Muscles

Epsom salt is known to soothe sore muscles because it contains magnesium. This invigorating combination of Epsom salt with shea butter and essential oils is sure to help remove stiffness and tension from your hard-working body.

Makes: 12 ounces

Ingredients

⅓ cup raw shea butter

¼ cup olive oil

½ teaspoon tangerine essential oil

20 drops lavender essential oil

20 drops eucalyptus essential oil

1 cup Epsom salts

Directions

Place the shea butter in a heatproof bowl and melt it in the microwave at 50% power.

Add the olive oil and mix.

Add the essential oils one at a time, mixing after each addition.

Pour in the Epsom salts and mix thoroughly.

To use, massage the scrub over sore muscles and rinse off. A scoop may be added to bathwater for a soothing soak.

Anti-Cellulite Scrub

Take your basic coffee scrub to a higher level by adding sugar for better stimulation. This improves circulation, and with coffee's anti-cellulite and tightening effects, you'll have softer, smoother, younger-looking skin. The vanilla has anti-inflammatory properties, while its aroma helps you to relax.

Makes: 8 ounces

Ingredients ¼ cup finely ground dry coffee ½ cup sugar

½ teaspoon natural vanilla extract 2 tablespoons coconut oil

2 tablespoons castor oil

Directions

Mix the coffee, sugar, and vanilla in a bowl. Gradually add the oils while mixing. Apply to problem areas and rub in a circular motion. Rinse with warm water.

SKIN CARE

Chapter 16 Coffee-Based and for Oily Skin Body Scrubs

Ah, yes. The benefits of a warm cup of coffee in the morning. You can't do anything without it. Coffee's health benefits on your interior are incredible: it provides antioxidants that work from the inside to reduce free radicals in your skin—thus preventing wrinkles and cancer-causing cells.

Do-it-yourself body scrubs with coffee ground bases also provide miraculous benefits to your exterior.

When coffee and caffeine are found in facial scrubs, they can reduce the appearance of puffy, tired eyes. These scrubs cut down on skin cell inflammation and swelling, thus working to heal your cells by decreasing their interior free radicals. The reduction of free radicals allows your facial cells to have more malleable cell membranes. Malleable cell membranes work to introduce more nutrients and moisture into the cells and expel all waste. Damaged, free radical-laden cells cannot reduce this waste and therefore simply die, leaving wrinkles in their place.

Furthermore, coffee ground scrubs can temporarily decrease cellulite. The caffeine-laden scrubs bring water to the cellulite, thus allowing the skin to look full. Unfortunately, this technique only brings temporary relief: anywhere from three to six hours. If you're on your way to the beach, look to these coffee scrubs for immediate, brief cellulite reduction.

Coffee ground scrubs bring great exfoliation to your skin, as well. It reduces the dry, dead cells and allows the new skin cells to reveal themselves. This allows a fresh, youthful look on your face.

Brown Sugar Caffeine-Boosting Body Scrub

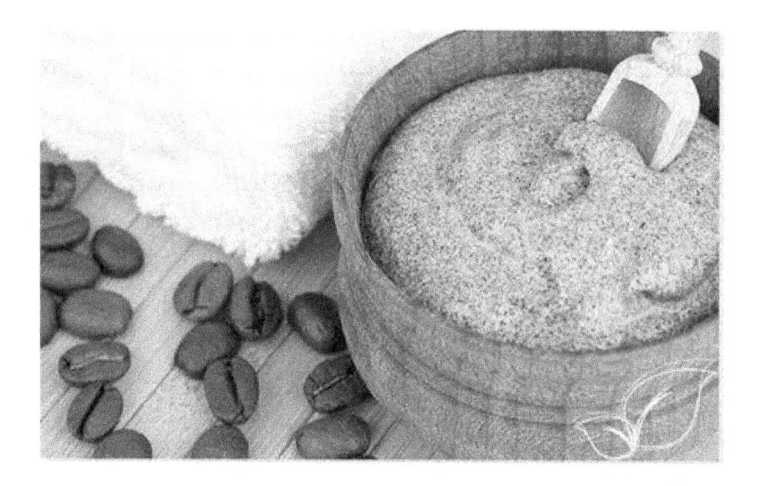

Ingredients:

1 cup coffee grounds

½ cup white sugar

1 cup coconut oil

Directions:

Mix your ingredients together—either thoroughly with a whisk or in a food processor. Apply the scrub to damp skin, adding a few drops of water in order to allow proper spreading. Allow it to remain on your body for two to three minutes. Prior to rinsing off in the shower, try to remove as much of the grounds gently with a towel. You don't want to clog up your shower! Enjoy your exfoliated, fresh skin.

Cuppa-Olive Oil Facial Scrub

Ingredients:

4 tbsp. olive oil

6 tbsp. coffee grounds

Directions:

Mix your ingredients together utilizing a whisk or a food processor. The product should look like a coarse, dirt-heavy mud. Apply a dollop of the mixture to your already damp face. Scrub gently for two to three minutes and rinse with warm water. View your result: a youthful, fresh-looking face.

Cinnamon Coconut Coffee Body Scrub

Note: This recipe contains cinnamon. Cinnamon rids the exterior skin of bacteria while also boosting blood flow to the dermis. This boost in blood flow rejuvenates the new cell creation many levels below the surface, allowing your future surface skin cells to glow with youthful, nutrient-rich shine.

Ingredients: ½ cup coffee grounds ½ cup coconut palm sugar

¼ cup coconut oil 1 tsp. ground cinnamon

Directions:

Mix the coffee grounds, coconut palm sugar, coconut oil, and ground cinnamon together well with either a spoon or a food processor. The result should be a coarse, muddy product. Utilize a handful with a few drops of water to cover your entire body. Scrub each area for approximately two minutes prior to rinsing off with warm water. You will be in awe at the sheer exfoliating power of coconut and coffee grounds.

Vanilla Latte Body Scrub

Note: Vanilla is utilized in several over-the-counter skin scrubs. It contains B-vitamins niacin, B6, thiamin, and pantothenic acid. These vitamins maintain a healthy glow and work to create future, healthy cells in the skin layers below.

Ingredients:

½ cup coffee grounds

½ cup organic white sugar

2 tbsp. coconut oil

2 tbsp. castor oil

½ tsp. vanilla extract

Directions:

Pour the coffee grounds, sugar, and vanilla in a medium bowl and mix well. Next, pour in the castor oil and the coconut oil. The desired consistency should be a bit like coarse mud. Upon application, utilize a few drops of water in order to scrub yourself well. Scrub for two to three minutes on your body. Do not utilize on your face because white sugar is far too coarse for delicate skin. Remember: this recipe is especially beneficial to rid yourself—temporarily—of cellulite.

Oily skin leads to acne. And oily skin is on the rise across the country—leading to increased acne attacks and worldwide discomfort. What is the cause of oily, acne-prone skin?

1. Genetics.

If your parents produce extra oil in their skin sebaceous glands, you do, as well. Extra oil is likely to clog your pores, and clogged pores, of course, lead to acne breakouts.

2. Skin care product over-usage.

The constant beauty-regiment you've maintained for several years could leave you extra-oily and extra-prone to acne. These beauty-regiments were meant to reduce your wrinkles or clear your skin; in reality, they're doing just the opposite in pummeling your skin with too much moisture.

3. Stress.

When your body is stressed, you create extra androgen hormones. These hormones force your body to create more skin oils. Afterwards, your body's pores are more apt to clog.

4. Sun-Tanning

Initially, sun-tanning rips the oils from your skin as it dries it out. However, when your body realizes its devoid of oils, it creates an instate injury response. The sebaceous glands go into oil-overdrive.

Look to the following recipes to reduce your face's oils and halt clogged pores.

Lemon Juice And Aspirin Anti-Acne Face Mask

Note: This recipe contains aspirin. Aspirin contains salicylic acid, an acid that helps regulate your skin's oils and heals your acne.

Ingredients:

4 aspirin

1 lemon

1 tsp. baking soda

Directions:

Crush the aspirin with a coffee cup or a rolling pin. You can add more aspirin if your oily or acne-prone coverage is large. Next, place the aspirin grounds in a small bowl. Squeeze lemon juice into the bowl and stir. The consistency should be like a paste. You can add more lemon as you stir.

Apply the aspirin mask to your face or just in the desired spots. Allow the mask to dry. This should take about fifteen minutes. Remove the mask by dipping a wet washcloth in baking soda and rubbing it lightly, in a circular motion, around your face.

Anti-Oil And Anti-Acne Oatmeal Face Mask

Ingredients:

¼ cup boiling water

1/3 cup oatmeal

1 large onion

½ tsp. honey

Directions:

Bring ¼ cup of water to a boil and pour it over the oatmeal in a bowl. Allow the oatmeal to steep for five minutes. While you're waiting, quarter the onion and place it all in the food processor. Make a puree. Next, add the pureed onion and the honey to the oatmeal paste and stir. Add more honey if the mask is thin.

While the mask is still warm, apply on your face. Leave it on for ten to fifteen minutes. The mask should harden. Remove the mask with a warm, wet washcloth.

Turmeric Indian Face Mask

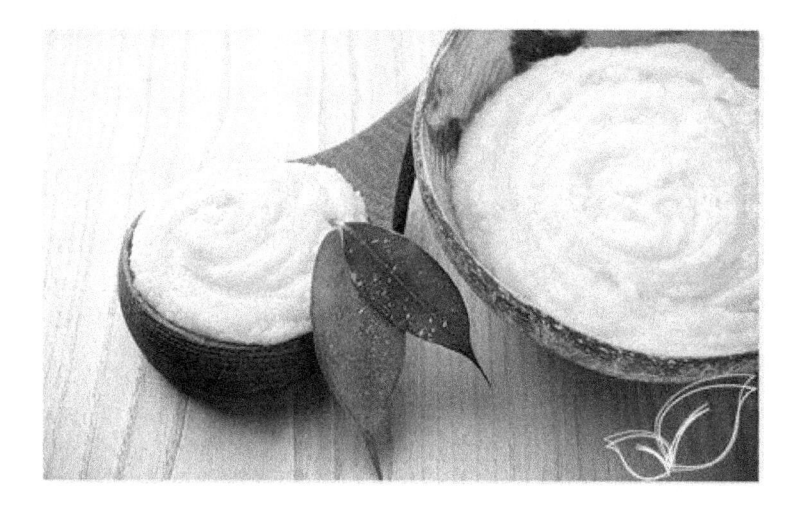

Note: Turmeric is an Indian spice found in many Indian foods. Indian women utilize it to give them a healthy, facial glow as well. It brightens the face and works with the yogurt and lemon juice to rejuvenate your facial cells and strip away some of those acne-causing oils.

Note: Turmeric may stain fair skin. The stain lasts only a few hours.

Ingredients: 2 tbsp. flour ¼ tsp. turmeric powder ¼ cup plain yogurt

2-3 drops lemon juice 2-3 drops honey

Directions:

Bring the flour and the turmeric powder together in a medium-sized bowl. Add the drops of lemon juice and stir slowly. Begin to add the yogurt just a bit at a time. A creamy paste should form.

Apply the turmeric mask to your face and allow it to sit for approximately twenty minutes. Choose an old, clean washcloth to wipe your face off with; turmeric will stain your nice washcloths.

Basic Clay Face Mask

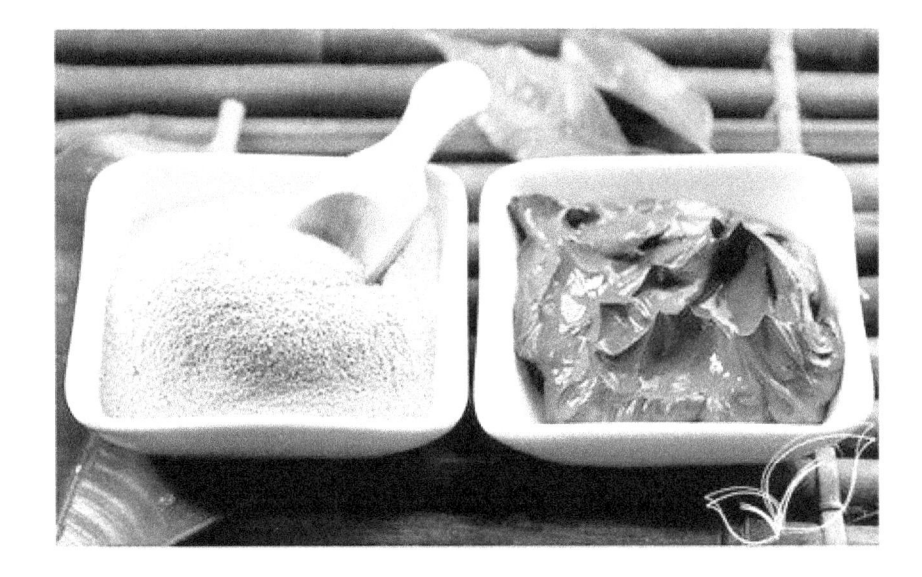

Note: Find basic bentonite clay from any local health food store.

Ingredients:Bentonite clay from health food store 1 tbsp. honey water

optional: essential oil of your choice

Directions:

The Bentonite clay comes in powder form at the store. Add two parts water to one-part clay depending on the amount of clay mask you'd like to make. It does store in the refrigerator rather well for up to five days. Mix the clay and water together and add the honey. If you'd like to add a bit of essential oil for a fresh, floral feeling, you can. This step is optional. Place the clay mask on your face and allow it to harden. This should take about fifteen minutes. Afterwards, rinse the mask off with a warm washcloth. Reap the rewards of this clay-oriented mask that helps you reduce the oils on your face and works to eliminate acne.

Chapter 17 Oatmeal-Based Body Scrub Recipes

Basic Oatmeal Scrub

A way to soothe the skin and exfoliate at the same time.

Ingredients:

Oatmeal

Warm water

Directions:

Let water warm.

Blend with oats and make paste.

Baking Soda & Oatmeal Scrub

Baking soda provides cleansing properties.

Ingredients:

2 tablespoons Oatmeal

1 teaspoon Baking soda

Directions:

Blend ingredients together.

If necessary, place in separate container for storage.

Almonds, Honey, Oatmeal And Apple Cider Vinegar Body Scrub

Honey works to moisturize. The vinegar works as an astringent and restores balance.

Ingredients:

8 tablespoons of organic Oatmeal

1 tablespoon of Apple cider Vinegar

1 tablespoon of organic Dark Honey

2 teaspoon of Almonds (finely ground)

Directions:

Heat honey in microwave.

Grind almonds in food processor

Blend ingredients together.

If necessary, place in separate container for storage.

Cucumber, Yogurt, Jojoba, Almond Oil And Oatmeal Scrub

Ingredients:

1/4 Cucumber (peeled)

2 tablespoons of organic yogurt (unflavored)

2 tablespoons of Oatmeal

1 teaspoon of Jojoba oil

1 teaspoon of Almond oil

Directions:

Blend ingredients together.

If necessary, place in separate container for storage.

Avocado, Almonds And Oatmeal Scrub

Ingredients:

1 cup of Organic Oatmeal 1 tablespoon of Almonds (coarsely ground)

1 ripe Avocado

Directions:

Peel the avocado

Blend ingredients together.

If necessary, place in separate container for storage.

Oatmeal, Cream Cheese And Lemon Juice Scrub

Ingredients:

2 tablespoons of Organic Oatmeal 1 tablespoon of Cream cheese

1 teaspoon of Lemon juice (fresh)

Directions:

Blend ingredients together.

If necessary, place in separate container for storage.

Almonds, Orange Peels And Oatmeal Scrub

Ingredients:

1 cup of Orange peels (dried)

1 cup of Organic Oatmeal 2 tablespoons of Almonds (finely ground)

1 teaspoon of sweet Orange essential oil

Directions:

Blend ingredients together.

If necessary, place in separate container for storage.

Lavender, Almond, Cornstarch, Chamomile And Oatmeal Body Scrub

Ingredients:

1/4 cup of Almonds

4 tablespoons of Organic Oatmeal

1 tablespoon of Cornstarch

1 tablespoon of dried Chamomile flowers (crushed)

2 teaspoons of Lavender essential oil

Directions:

Blend ingredients together.

If necessary, place in separate container for storage.

Cranberries, Coconut, Brown Sugar, Almond, Olive Oil And Oatmeal Body Scrub

Berries in this recipe help to exfoliate. The oils provide moisture.

Ingredients:

1/2 cup of Cranberries

4 tablespoons of Organic Oatmeal

2 tablespoons of Coconut oil

2 tablespoons of Sugar (Brown)

1 tablespoon of Almond oil

1 tablespoon of Olive oil

Directions:

Blend ingredients together.

If necessary, place in separate container for storage.

Fuller's Earth, Lavender, Almond, Mint, Oatmeal And Chamomile Body Scrub

Works great on skin that is oily.

Ingredients:

1 cup of Organic Oatmeal 4 tablespoons of Almonds (finely grounded)

2 teaspoons of dried Lavender (crushed)

1 teaspoon of dried peppermint (crushed)

1 teaspoon of dried Chamomile flowers (crushed)

Fuller's Earth

Directions:

Blend ingredients together, leaving Fuller's Earth out.

Blend a ratio of 2 tablespoons mix and 1 tablespoon Fuller's Earth to make paste when ready to use.

If necessary, place in separate container for storage.

Butternut Squash And Oatmeal Scrub

Ingredients: 1 Tablespoon Rolled Oats

1 Tablespoon Almonds (Slivered or Whole)

1 Tablespoon Squash Seeds, or Pepitas, or Sunflower Seeds

2 Teaspoons Water (Oily Skin), or Milk (Normal Skin), or Heavy Cream (Dry Skin)

2 Teaspoons Cooked Butternut Squash Pinch of Cinnamon

Directions:

In processor, grind nuts.Add with milk and everything but squash and cinnamonBlend all ingredients together.

If necessary, place in separate container for storage.

Pumpkin Spice Scrub

Ingredients:

3/4 cup of cane sugar

3 Tablespoons of almond oil

3 Tablespoons of organic oats (plain)

1 Tablespoon of pumpkin puree

1 teaspoon of cinnamon (grounded)

1/2 teaspoon of nutmeg (grounded)

4 drops of ylang-ylang essential oil

1 drop of ginger essential oil

1 drop of clove essential oil

Directions:

Blend ingredients together. Use food processor for convenience.

If necessary, place in separate container for storage.

Oatmeal Honey Scrub Recipe:

Ingredients:

Two parts oatmeal

One-part honey

One-part sweet almond oil

Directions:

Blend ingredients together.

If necessary, place in separate container for storage.

Coconut Oatmeal Scrub

Ingredients:

1 1/2 cup Oatmeal

1/2 cup Organic Coconut Oil

1 tsp vanilla extract

1 tsp honey

1 tsp brown sugar

Directions:

Blend ingredients together.

If necessary, place in separate container for storage.

Oatmeal Almond Body Scrub

Ingredients:

2/3 cup almonds {whole, slivers, slices, whatever you have}

2/3 cup oatmeal

1/2 cup brown sugar

1/4 cup olive oil

1/4 cup coconut oil

2 Tbsp honey

1 tsp vanilla

Directions:

Blend ingredients together.

If necessary, place in separate container for storage

SKIN CARE

Chapter 18 Salt and Sugar-Free Body Scrubs

Ran out of salt and sugar in the kitchen? Don't fret. It is still possible to create a luscious body scrub without these two popular ingredients. You just need something coarse to replace them such as oatmeal, almond meal or nuts. Will the result still be as effective without these two basic ingredients? The answer is yes, and for some people, even more favorable. Everyone has different types of skin. Therefore, some people yield more positive results to body scrubs that contain other ingredients such as oatmeal, almonds and other fruits and vegetables. Check out some of the recipes below, try them out and see if these will also work for you. These recipes are best for all types of skin.

Here are some salt and sugar free body scrub recipes your body will surely love!

Oatmeal Chamomile Scrub

Ingredients: 4 tablespoons ground almonds, 1 tablespoon cornstarch, 4 tablespoons oatmeal, 1 tablespoon chamomile flowers, 2 tablespoons sweet almond oil, and 5 drops lavender extract

Directions: Place the ground almonds, cornstarch and oatmeal in a spice grinder or blender. Add the chamomile flowers and process well. Mix in the sweet almond oil and lavender extract. Stir well. To use, get a handful of the scrub and add several drops of water. Massage on damp skin for several minutes and wash off with warm water.

Main ingredient: ground almonds and chamomile flowers

Almonds are rich in phytochemicals that treat pimples, acne, and other skin conditions. It also reduces sebum production and prevents overly oily skin. Chamomile's anti-inflammatory and antiseptic properties soothe skin redness and swelling brought upon by acne, eczema, and minor burns.

Firming Scrub

Ingredients: 2 egg whites, 2 bay leaves, 1 celery stalk, ½ cup unpeeled cucumber slices, ¼ cup wheat germ, ½ cup hearts of palm (chopped), ¼ cup full-fat powdered milk, ¼ unpeeled russet potato slices, 1 teaspoon mint leaves, 1 teaspoon coconut extract, and 1 teaspoon vanilla extract

Ingredients: Place all the ingredients in a blender. Process until all the contents takes on a thick consistency. Apply all over the body and massage for several minutes. Leave on for 20 minutes before rinsing with lukewarm water.

Main ingredient: russet potato, and celery

Russet potatoes naturally brighten the skin's complexion, refresh tired skin, remove dark spots, and nourish very dry skin. It also prevents acne, heal insect stings and bites, and soothe minor burns. Celery contains powerful antioxidants that delay skin aging, protect from free radical damage, and hydrates from the inside out. It also maintains the skin luminosity and elasticity.

Honey Wheat Germ Scrub

Ingredients: 2 tablespoons clear honey, 1 tablespoon wheat germ, 1 teaspoon sunflower oil, and 1 teaspoon fresh lemon juice

Directions: In small bowl, combine the wheat germ and the honey. Add the sunflower oil and lemon juice to the mixture. Stir well. Scrub on damp skin for several minutes. Rinse thoroughly.

Main ingredient: wheat germ

Wheat germ is rich in zinc which helps in skin cell production. It also contains anti-inflammatory properties that stop symptoms of eczema and other skin diseases and lessen acne swelling.

Almond Meal Scrub

Ingredients: ½ cup ground almond meal, 1/2 cup oats (finely ground oats), and rosewater

Directions: Place the oats and almonds in the blender. Process them until well-combined. Transfer into a small bowl. Gently pour in the rosewater drop by drop until a paste is formed. Apply on damp skin and massage for several minute. Leave on skin for 30 minutes before rinsing.

Main ingredient: almond meal

Almond meal helps smoothen and soften the skin and removes dead skin cells. It also reduces swelling and clarifies skin complexion.

Grapefruit And Oatmeal Body Scrub

Ingredients: 1 fresh grapefruit, 2 tablespoons oatmeal

Directions: Squeeze out the pulp and juice of the grapefruit and put it in a bowl. Add in the oatmeal and mix until it turns into a smooth paste. You can add in more oatmeal or juice in order to get the consistency you desire. Scrub the paste-like mixture on the face and on the body. Leave on for a few minutes before rinsing.

Main ingredient: grapefruit, oatmeal

The grapefruit contains citrus that helps stimulate the skin and aids in exfoliation. The coarseness of the oatmeal provides a gentle exfoliation while hydrating the skin.

Baking Soda And Oatmeal Scrub

Ingredients: 2 heaping tablespoons of oatmeal, 1 teaspoon of baking soda, water

Directions: Mix the two ingredients together. Gradually add in small amounts of water until the mixture turns into a sticky paste. This recipe will only make a small amount of scrub. Double or triple the ingredients if you desire to make more. Massage the mixture in the face and body in a circular motion. Let it sit for a few minutes before rinsing.

Main ingredient: Baking soda

Baking soda is ideal for exfoliation because it is not too coarse and therefore helps to exfoliate the top layer of the dead skin cells gently. It is also safe to use even on sensitive skin.

Apple Cider Oatmeal Scrub

Ingredients: 8 tablespoons oatmeal, 1 tablespoon apple cider, 1 tablespoon dark organic honey, 2 teaspoons ground almonds

Directions: Warm the honey until it becomes a little runny or watery, but not too hot so it won't burn. Place the melted honey in a bowl and add in all the other ingredients. Mix everything until it turns into a smooth paste. Rub the mixture on the skin in a circular motion and leave on for 10 to 15 minutes. Rinse with alternating warm and cold water but end it in a splash of cold water to close the pores.

Main ingredient: apple cider

Apple cider vinegar has long been used for treating warts, acne and other skin problems. It also has antibacterial properties that can help rid the skin of common problems associated with bacterial infection.

Cucumber Yogurt Scrub

Ingredients: ¼ medium peeled cucumber, 2 tablespoons plain unflavored yogurt (with active cultures), 2 tablespoons oatmeal, 1 teaspoon jojoba, 1 teaspoon sweet almond oil

Directions: Cut the cucumber into small pieces and put them in a blender or food processor to liquefy. Add in the rest of the ingredients to the food processor or blender and whisk until the mixture turns into a smooth paste. Rub onto body and face in a circular motion then rinse with alternating warm and cold water.

Main ingredient: cucumber, yogurt

Cucumber is best known for reducing eye bags and removing dark circles under the eye. Other benefits on skin include treating sunburn, tightening pores, and reducing freckles. Yogurt, when eaten is packed with nutrients such as zinc, calcium and B-vitamins. But it also helps tighten skin pores and remove acne.

Avocado-Almond Scrub

Ingredients: 1 cup oatmeal, 1 tablespoon ground Almonds, 1 ripe avocado (peeled)

Directions: Mix the oatmeal and almonds and then set aside. Mash the peeled avocado to a pulp. Using a clean washcloth, grab some of the avocado pulp then dip it in the almond and oatmeal mixture. Rub onto skin in a circular motion to exfoliate. Rinse thoroughly and tone and moisturize afterwards.

Main ingredient: avocado

Avocado is rich in antioxidants plus vitamins A and C. It is used to moisturize not only the skin but also the hair.

Chapter 19 Fruit and Coffee-Based Scrub Recipes

Orange Sugar Scrub

Ingredients:

¾ cup sugar (plus 1-2tbsp more)

4 drops orange essential oil

¼ cup coconut oil (melted)

1 tbsp dried orange peel (coarsely grinded)

¼ cup olive oil

Instructions:

Mix all ingredients together and place it in a clean container.

If mixture is too dry, add some more oil. If too oily, add a little more sugar.

Lime Margarita Mousse Scrub

Ingredients:

2 drops lemon essential oil 4 drops lime essential oil

½ tsp lime or lemon juice 2 tsp virgin coconut oil

1½ tsp salt 2 tsp white sugar

10 drops kukui nut oil, sweet almond oil or apricot kernel oil

Instructions:

Combine the ingredients well. (The salt will stay nice and grainy, but the sugar will mostly dissolve in the lime juice)

Apply to body.

Lemon & Coconut Milk Scrub

Ingredients:

¼ cup coconut oil 2 tbsp coconut milk ¼ cup sugar 1 tbsp lemon zest

1 tsp lemon juice

Instructions:

In a double boiler, melt the coconut oil over low heat 15- 20 seconds.

Add sugar and coconut milk, mixing until sugar is well coated.

Add lemon zest and lemon juice until all ingredients are thoroughly combined. Store in a glass jar.

Coffee Sugar Scrub

Ingredients:

½ cup used ground coffee

½ cup ground coffee

½ cup coconut oil

1 cup sugar

1 tsp cinnamon

1 tsp vegetable glycerin (for extra moisturizer)

Instructions:

Pour coffee grounds and sugar into a medium sized bowl.

Stir in coconut oil or more if you prefer a wet consistency.

Now add cinnamon, mix and place in the jar.

Solid Shea Butter Cube

Ingredients:

4 oz refined Shea butter

2.5 oz Shea butter soap base 2 tbsp fractionated coconut oil

16 oz white sugar

½ tbsp essential oils of choice

Pinch of mica (optional)

Instructions:

Melt soap base and Shea butter and stir. Add the fractionated coconut oil and essential oils and stir.

Pour the sugar into the soap/ Shea mixture, mixing well. Scoop into mold and use a spatula to level. Refrigerate until solidified.

Remove the scrub gently from the molds. Remove plastic wrap from scrub. Cut the scrub into cubes with a Chef's knife.

Place cubes in an airtight jar until use.

Seedy Oatmeal Body Scrub

Ingredients:

1 handful coarse rolled oats   1 handful brown lentils

½ tsp jojoba oil   ½ tsp carrot oil

Water

Instructions:

Blend the lentils in a blender until it is a coarse powder.

Add the rolled oats and blend to make powder. Add the oils and then process again.

Slowly add water until mixture becomes a thick paste. Spoon into a container.

Organic Citrus Sugar Scrub

Ingredients:

1 small lime   1 small lemon   ½ cup coconut oil   1 cup pure cane sugar

1 teaspoon peppermint essential oil

Mint Leaves, lemon & lime peels (optional)

Instructions:

Mix together the oil and moist ingredients.

Add the sugar. If using, add the lime and lemon peels as a garnish.

Stir, bottle and use within 3 months.

Coconut Oatmeal Scrub

Ingredients:

½ cup organic coconut oil   1½ cup oatmeal   1 tsp brown sugar

1 tsp vanilla extract   1 tsp honey

Instructions:

In a food processor, ground oatmeal and place in a bowl.

Add brown sugar to finely ground oatmeal and then mix.

Pour vanilla, coconut oil and honey to the oatmeal and then mix until thoroughly combined.

Store in an airtight container.

Cucumber Oatmeal Scrub

Ingredients:

1 cucumber (2 tbsp cucumber paste)   1tsp rosehip oil   1 teaspoon argan oil

2 tbsp oatmeal   1 tbsp milk

Instructions:

Blend cucumber in the blender to make a paste.

Add 2 tablespoon of the blended cucumber with the rest of the ingredients, mixing well.

Leave for about 5 minutes until oatmeal gets soft.

Use and discard leftover.

Coffee Morning Scrub

Ingredients:

2 tbsp freshly ground coffee   3 tbsp whole milk or heavy cream

2 tbsp cocoa powder   1 tbsp honey

Instructions:

Mix all together and apply lightly to face.

Leave for 15-20 minutes.

Remove with warm wash cloth.

Anti-Cellulite Coffee Scrub

Ingredients:

½ cup ground coffee

1½ cup turbinado sugar

½ cup grape seed oil

½ cup jojoba oil

1 tsp vitamin E

1 tsp vanilla extract

1 tsp sage essential oil

Instructions:

Mix all ingredients well

Transfer the now gritty paste to an airtight container using a spoon

Label, date and store in a cool place.

Use scrub within 3 months.

Cup Of Joe Scrub

Ingredients:

6 tbsp coffee grounds

1/3 cup brown sugar

4 tbsp olive oil

Instructions:

Mix the two ingredients together until it looks like a coarse mud. (The coffee grounds have to be very fine as they will be rubbed onto the skin. If necessary, put them through a coffee grinder twice)

Transfer to a container, refrigerate or store at room temperature for 5-7 weeks.

Chapter 20 Additional Body Scrub Recipes

Purifying Body Scrub

Equipment Needed: Measuring Cup, Eye Dropper, Bowl, Stirring Spoon

Ingredients:

¾ of a Cup of Epsom salts

¼ of a Cup of baking soda

4 drops of grapefruit essential oil

Almond or jojoba oil

Directions:

Combine the first three ingredients into your bowl.

Begin slowly adding the Almond or Jojoba oil while stirring.

Add just enough of the oil to create a paste.

Note: This scrub should be applied to your body, not your face. Use "scrubbing" motion when applying, shower afterwards.

Peppermint Body Scrub

Equipment Needed: Measuring Cup, Measuring Spoon, Eye Dropper, Medium-Size Bowl, Fork, Wide-Mouth Jar w/ Lid

Ingredients:

¼ of a Cup of olive oil

1 tsp of pure vanilla extract

1 Cup of pure turbinado sugar

15 drops of peppermint essential oil

½ of a Cup of used coffee grounds from a freshly brewed pot

Directions:

Place all of the ingredients in your bowl.

Combine the ingredients thoroughly w/ fork.

Transfer to your jar.

Store in cool environment.

Shelf-life is up to two weeks, longer if placed in fridge.

Note: This scrub should be applied while showering. Take handfuls and apply in circular motions working from your feet upwards. Thoroughly rinse scrub from body. Use a body wash, dry yourself off, and apply a quality body lotion.

Star Anise Body Scrub

Equipment Needed: Measuring Cup, Bowl, Eye Dropper, Stirring Spoon

Ingredients:

½ of a Cup of coconut oil

½ of a Cup of brown sugar

6 drops of star anise essential oil

Directions:

Combine the ingredients into your bowl.

Stir thoroughly.

Note: Apply and massage the scrub into the skin while showering.

Mandarin Body Scrub

Equipment Needed: Measuring Cup, Eye Dropper, Bowl, Stirring Spoon, Jar w/ Lid

Ingredients: 1 Cup of white sugar ⅓ of a Cup of olive oil

10 drops of mandarin-scented essential oil

Directions:

Combine the sugar and oil in your bowl.

Mix well.

Now add the Essential oil.

Stir thoroughly.

Transfer to jar & cover.

Citrus-Salt Body Scrub

Equipment Needed: Measuring Cup, Measuring Spoon, Grater, Medium-Size Bowl, Airtight Container

Ingredients: ½ of a Cup of sea salt ½ of a Cup of sweet almond oil

½ of a tsp of lemon zest ½ of a tsp of orange zest Orange

Directions:

Begin by grating your orange.

Place the zest into your bowl.

Add-in the rest of the ingredients.

Stir thoroughly.

Transfer to container & store in cool/dry environment.

Note: Use your finger to mix-up the ingredients before using. Apply to skin before entering the shower using a circular motion.

Ylang-Ylang Body Scrub

Equipment Needed: Measuring Cup, Eye Dropper, Bowl, Stirring Spoon

Ingredients:

½ of a Cup of coconut oil

½ of a Cup of brown sugar

8 drops of ylang-ylang essential oil

Directions:

Place ingredients into your bowl.

Thoroughly mix.

Note: Apply and massage into skin while showering.

Strawberry Belly & Breast Scrub

Equipment Needed: Blender, Measuring Spoons, Fork, Stirring Spoon, 2 Bowls, Spatula, Knife & Cutting Board

Ingredients:

12 ripe strawberries

2 Tbsp of cold-pressed avocado oil

3 Tbsp of distilled witch hazel solution

3 Tbsp of rice flour

1 tsp of aloe gel

Whole cucumber

Directions:

First take the strawberries and remove stems.

Using your knife remove any bad or white portions.

Place the berries in a bowl.

Mash with fork.

Put the cucumber into your blender.

Puree without removing skin or seeds.

Place the avocado oil & pureed cucumber into another bowl.

Stir thoroughly.

Now add-in the berries and witch hazel.

Take the flour & sprinkle it on top of the wet mixture.

Using your spatula, fold the flour into the wet ingredients

Finally, add the aloe & stir to create a paste.

Note: First spray-on a body mist beginning at your lower neck downward to your belly. After five minutes apply the scrub mixture to your upper chest, breasts and abdomen. Allow the scrub to remain on skin for fifteen minutes before rinsing. This scrub is rich in vitamins A, C, and E.

Cornmeal Thigh Scrub

Equipment Needed: Measuring Spoons, Eye Dropper, Paper Bag, Wooden Mallet, Food Processor, Sterile Jar w/ Lid, Bowl, Stirring Spoon

Ingredients:

1 small avocado pit

4 Tbsp of cornmeal

2 tsp of aloe gel

1 Tbsp of cold-pressed grape seed oil

6 drops of juniper essential oil

6 drops of lemon essential oil

Directions:

Begin the recipe by placing the avocado pit into the paper bag.

Use the mallet to crush the pit.

Place the pit into your processor.

Grind until the consistency is similar to a meal.

Add-in the cornmeal & mix thoroughly.

Transfer to jar and seal.

Now put the grape seed, aloe, juniper and lemon oils in your bowl.

Take two teaspoons of the avocado/cornmeal mixture on top of the wet ingredients.

Stir.

Note: Mist legs before applying scrub. Use circular motions when applying the mixture. Allow the scrub to remain on your skin for fifteen minutes before rinsing.

Peppermint Candy Cane Sugar Scrub

Equipment Needed: Measuring Cup, Eye Dropper, Mixing Bowl, 2 Containers, Stirring Spoon, Large Piece Of Paper, Jar w/ Lid

Ingredients:

2 Cups of granulated sugar

¼ to ⅓ of a Cup of Almond or Coconut oil

3 drops of Peppermint Essential oil.

Coloring

Directions:

Place the sugar in your mixing bowl.

Gradually begin adding the coconut or almond oil.

Stir until your consistency is soft & smooth.

Now add-in the Essential oil.

Stir.

Divide the mixture between the two containers.

Add some coloring into one of the containers.

Take the piece of paper and form it into a funnel.

Place the funnel into the jar.

Begin building layers of white & colored scrub.

Pour an amount of the colored scrub into the jar.

Press-down the mixture inside the jar to make it even.

Now pour an equal amount of colored scrub.

Press-down the mixture just as you did the first layer.

Repeat the process until either the jar is full, or you have used-up the mixture.

Glycerin, Coconut And Sweet Orange Oil Salt Scrub

Equipment Needed: Measuring Spoons, Measuring Cup, Stirring Spoon, Scoop, Saucepan, Towel, Jar w/ Lid

Ingredients:

8 Tbsp of liquid Glycerin

½ of a Cup of Mineral Water

3 Cups of Table Salt

1 tsp of solid Coconut oil

½ of a tsp of sweet Orange oil

Directions:

Start this recipe by combining the glycerin, water & a Cup of the salt.

Stir until the all of the ingredients are completely dissolved.

Now take the remaining salt & begin stirring into the mixture.

Continue adding until you create a paste.

Put the coconut oil in your saucepan.

Place overheat and cook until the oil has melted.

Remove from the heat immediately so the oil doesn't overheat.

Begin to add the oil into the salt gradually.

Continue stirring until well-blended.

Now take the sweet orange oil & add to the mixture.

Using your scoop, transfer the mixture to the jar & apply lid.

Place in fridge and allow to thicken before using.

Note: When using the scrub, apply and massage into skin. The scrub is an exfoliate so be sure to wash off using warm and then cold water. Pat dry w/ towel, and then tone and add moisturizer.

Coconut Salt Scrub

Equipment Needed: Measuring Cup, Eye Dropper, Bowl, Stirring Spoon, Container w/ Lid

Ingredients:

1 Cup of salt

¼ of a Cup of coconut oil

¼ of a Cup of Vitamin E oil

3 to 4 drops of Essential oil

Directions:

Place the coconut oil, salt & Vitamin E oil in your bowl.

Now add the Essential oil.

Stir thoroughly.

Transfer to container & apply lid.

Chamomile, Aloe Vera, Castile Soap And Lavender Oil Salt Scrub

Equipment Needed: Measuring Spoons, Bowl, Stirring Spoon, Towel, And Jar w/ Lid

Ingredients:

6 Tbsp of Avocado oil

2 Tbsp of Aloe Vera gel

8 Tbsp of Castile soap

12 Tbsp of Dead Sea salt

1 Tsp of Lavender essential oil

1 Tbsp of crushed dried Chamomile flowers

Directions:

Combine all of the ingredients into your bowl

Stir until the mixture has the consistency of paste.

Transfer to jar and cover.

Note: Massage the scrub gently onto damp skin using a circular motion. This scrub is an exfoliate so be sure to rinse with warm and then cold water. Pat-dry with towel, use toner and then a moisturizer.

Rosemary And Peppermint Sea Salt Scrub

Equipment Needed: Measuring Cup, Eye Dropper, Saucepan, Stirring Spoon

Ingredients:

2 Cups of Coarse-grain sea salt 1 Cup of Olive Oil

¼ of an oz of Liquid glycerin soap

5 drops of Rosemary essential oil

5 drops of Peppermint essential oil

Directions:

Put the soap & oil in your saucepan.

Place overheat & warm.

Now stir-in the rosemary, salt & peppermint oils

Set to the side to cool.

Citrus Salt Scrub

Equipment Needed: Measuring Cup, Measuring Spoon, Saucepan, Large Bowl, Stirring Spoon, Airtight Container

Ingredients:

½ of a Cup of sea salt ½ of a Cup of coconut oil 1.5 tsp of citrus zest

Directions:

Put the coconut oil in your saucepan.

Place overheat & warm teaspoon

Now add the oil and the rest of the ingredients into the bowl.

Stir.

Transfer to your container.

Note: Be sure to store in a cool and dry environment.

Orange Salt Scrub

Equipment Needed: Measuring Spoon, Bowl, and Towel

Ingredients:

2 Tbsp of Sea salt

The juice of one-half of a fresh Orange

Directions:

After you have juiced the half orange & discarded the pulp, place the juice in a bowl.

Add the salt.

Stir together until your mixture has the consistency of paste.

Note: Use this scrub on your face and body. Use cold & then hot water to rinse. Pat dry with a towel and follow with a toner and moisturizer.

Chapter 21 Cleansing, Nourishing and Hydrating Exfoliants

Taking care of your skin has never been this easy. We'll use the healthy foods found right in your kitchen to make cleansing and restorative skin care products. From nutritious avocados to stimulating coffee grounds, you'll learn to take the simplest of ingredients and design your own exfoliants, scrubs and masks for cleansing, nourishing and hydrating your skin.

Nourishing Oat And Almond Exfoliant

The ingredients in this recipe have anti-inflammatory and antioxidant properties offering a soothing and hydrating treatment for all skin types. An excellent exfoliant for gently cleansing pores. Appropriate for body care as well as facial exfoliating.

Ingredients:

- 1 Tablespoon ground oats (choose gluten-free oats if you are gluten intolerant—this ensures you will avoid any possible systemic reaction from cross-contamination)
- 1 Tablespoon ground almonds
- ½ teaspoon rice flour
- 2 teaspoons warm water (or oil of your choice)

Directions: Combine and mix ingredients and wait until oats have slightly softened. Gently rub onto your skin in a circular motion for 1-2 minutes, avoiding the eye area. Leave on for 10 minutes and then rinse with warm water. Follow with a cold rinse.

Tip: Adding 2 cups of oats to your bath is useful in soothing and healing various skin conditions including dry, itchy skin.

Refreshing Lemon And Apple Exfoliant

Excellent for oily skin, lemon juice has alpha-hydroxy acids which enhance dead skin cell removal. As an exfoliant, lemon will help cleanse and refresh your skin. This recipe is specially formulated for facial skin use.

Ingredients:
- 1/8 cup lemon juice (for sensitive skin, pure aloe Vera juice may be used instead)
- ¼ cup apple juice
- ¼ cup water
- ¼ cup cane sugar (or jojoba beads for a gentler exfoliant)

Directions: Mix all ingredients in a glass jar or bowl until sugar is dissolved. Apply to skin with a cotton ball or clean, soft washcloth. Gently massaging in and rinse after 10 minutes with warm water.

Tip: Dab diluted lemon juice to the skin (and rinse with cold water after 5 minutes) to reduce skin discoloration and fade acne scarring.

Exhilarating Vanilla Coffee Scrub

Energize your skin with the antioxidant and anti-inflammatory properties of coffee. This scrub tones and firms your skin and can help reduce the appearance of cellulite. Though created to be used on any part of your body, this compound is gentle enough for your face.

Ingredients:

- 3 Tablespoons coffee grounds (can be from your freshly brewed pot!)
- 1 Tablespoon sugar (or jojoba beads for a gentler exfoliant)
- 2 Tablespoons almond oil (or other oil of your choice)
- ¼ teaspoon of vanilla extract

Directions: Mix ingredients together and massage into desired skin area. Leave on for 10 minutes and rinse with warm water. Pat dry. This can be stored in the refrigerator for a few months.

Tip: You can use cotton pads to soak up any leftover, cooled, brewed coffee and place under your eyes for 20 minutes to help reduce dark circles and puffiness.

Restorative Lavender Sugar Scrub

A soothing scrub suitable for all skin types (mainly dry or sensitive skin), this treatment also makes for a luxurious and relaxing bedtime routine.

Ingredients:

- ¼ cup sugar (or jojoba beads for a gentler exfoliant)
- ½ cup coconut oil (or other oil of your choice)
- 2-3 sprigs of dried lavender
- 4 drops of lavender pure essential oil

Directions: Separate dried lavender buds from sprigs. Place buds and other ingredients into a glass jar or bowl and mix. Rub a small amount onto desired area, especially effective for hands and feet. Let it set for 5 minutes before rinsing off with warm water and patting dry. This recipe stores well for several months in the refrigerator.

Tip: Lavender pure essential oil helps with bee stings and insect bites by reducing itching or swelling.

Maple Tangerine Peel Treatment

Rich in antioxidants and vitamins A and C, this tangerine-based mask brings about silky skin and a refreshed feel. Works well on dry patches or irritated skin.

Ingredients:

- 2 tablespoons ground and dried tangerine peel (peel can be dried in oven at lowest heat for an hour or on tray for a few days on the counter)
- 1 teaspoon ground flax seed
- 1 teaspoon maple syrup
- 1 teaspoon water
- 1 teaspoon coconut oil (almond oil will also work nicely)

Directions: Mix all ingredients together, gently apply to desired skin area (also safe for facial application) and leave on for 10 minutes. Rinse with warm water and pat dry.

Tip: Consuming ground flax seeds with their high content of vitamin E and omega-3 fatty acids nourishes hair follicles and lessens hair loss.

Softening Avocado Facial Mask

For nourishing and hydrating dry skin, it's hard to beat nutrient-packed avocados. Its natural oils include vitamin E oil which leaves your skin feeling silky smooth. In combination with vitamin A rich carrots, this formula acts as an excellent antiseptic as well.

Ingredients:

- ½ ripe avocado mashed
- 2 Tablespoons cooked, mashed and cooled carrot
- 1 Tablespoon olive oil (more oil may be added for dryer skin)
- A few drops of lemon juice

Directions: Mix all ingredients together and rub onto face in circular motions. Leave on for 15 minutes. Follow with a warm water rinse, then a cool rinse and pat dry.

Tip: Carrots with their high content of antioxidants provides anti-aging benefits. A mashed carrot mask may also be used on its own.

Turmeric Banana Sunshine Mask

This powerful anti-aging facial remedy is packed with antioxidants, vitamins and minerals, and will leave the skin feeling firm and radiant. Turmeric contains antibacterial, antifungal and anti-inflammatory properties making for an effective acne treatment. This recipe is suitable for all skin types.

Ingredients:
- 1 small banana
- 1 teaspoon of powdered turmeric
- 1 Tablespoon coconut cream (or plain coconut yoghurt)

Directions: Place banana into a bowl and mash well with a fork. Add coconut cream and turmeric powder. Mix until smooth. Apply mixture onto face and leave for up to 20 minutes. Rinse with warm water and pat dry. Take caution not to stain your clothes or towels!

Tip: Turmeric may be added to your natural shampoo products to reduce dandruff and to inhibit hair loss.

Sweet Cinnamon Lip Scrub

Using brown sugar and spicy cinnamon, this homemade formula is a delicious way to exfoliate dry skin and plump up your pout.

Ingredients:

- ¼ cup brown sugar
- 1 Tablespoon almond oil
- 1 teaspoon cinnamon powder

Directions: Mix together all ingredients and apply to your lips. Scrub gently in circular motions with your fingertips and leave on for 5-10 minutes. Rinse with warm water and follow with an oil based lip balm. This may be stored in the refrigerator for several weeks.

Tip: Cinnamon inhibits bacterial growth and makes an excellent preservative for your homemade body care products.

These luscious exfoliants, scrubs and masks are made to be an integral part of a total body care system, created by you with the purest of ingredients. They are most effective when followed by a rich and nourishing body butter, balm or lotion.

Conclusion

Shampoo, deodorants and moisturizers fill the medicine cabinets in just about every home in America. You probably spend a decent percentage of your weekly grocery budget on these and similar items and don't think twice about it because they are a necessity. But let me ask you something. Would you eat these products? Of course not! They are full of chemicals and unsafe materials. But by putting them on your body, you are essentially doing just that. You are consuming them. The chemicals in these products gain full access to your body when you apply them. They are able to penetrate your skin and enter the bloodstream when used as recommended by the companies that produce them.

These products can wreak havoc on your skin and overall health. Allergic reactions are common and skin irritation is not unheard of. Sometimes these chemicals can be carcinogens and cause some serious problems to organs, such as the liver and kidneys. Even the heart can be affected by these toxic synthetics put in your body care products.

Some of the more common chemicals found in bath and body products include several different forms of parabens. These are notorious for causing allergic skin reactions. They are highly toxic but favored by companies due to their low price and ability to extend the shelf life of a product. Almost every product will have fragrance listed as an ingredient, which is a blanket term for hundreds of different combinations of synthetic ingredients that can cause headaches, dizziness and rashes.

Mineral oil is a common ingredient that sounds safe, but when applied causes a barrier over the skin that slows down the development of new and healthy cells. It can also cause acne because it traps any bacteria that was on your skin before you applied it. Propylene glycol, found in shampoo and bubble bath, has been linked to kidney damage and abnormalities of the liver. Next time you pick up your conditioner or favorite body cream, take a moment to read the ingredients. Chances are, you will find one of the dangerous chemicals just mentioned.

So, what can you do to avoid the negative side effects of these chemicals? We are not suggesting that you stop bathing or give up your favorite beauty routines. Here, you are provided with recipes that will enable you to make all of your favorite bath and beauty products right in your own home. You will know every ingredient that goes into each product and will no longer have to worry about what you are putting in your body. These ingredients are easily accessible and won't break the bank. The most common ingredients used in homemade bath products are essential oils, carrier oils, herbs and other natural supplements.

Essential oils are concentrated liquids derived from plants, including leaves, flowers, roots and trees. They are made by extracting the liquid from the solid leaf or flower of the plant, usually by steam or pure expression. Essential oils are popular for their use in aromatherapy, or the use of certain fragrances to improve emotions and state of mind. While this will not be your main motivation for mixing up these products, it is a great extra perk. There are countless varieties of oils and all have different healing properties.

One of their best qualities is that they create an environment where bacteria and viruses find it difficult to live. They are great for the immune system and encourage healthy cell development. Because of the direct concentration of these oils, they will usually need to be diluted in order to be used safely. For this reason, it is not recommended that they be used by pregnant women or people with certain conditions, like epilepsy.

If you are unsure if you should be using these oils, consult with your doctor. If you are using essential oils, always do a spot test on your arm to make sure that there will not be a reaction. Simply take one drop of oil mixed with fifteen drops of carrier oil. Place a small amount on the skin. If there is no redness or irritation after twelve hours, the oil is safe for you to use. Investigate the company that you plan on purchasing your essential oils from.

Unfortunately, this market is not nationally regulated, and it is up to you to make sure that you are purchasing high quality ingredients. It is preferred that the oils be made from organic plants. This will ensure that your oil will be pesticide and chemical free.

A carrier oil is needed to dilute the essential oils enough to be safely used, since some oils can be very dangerous if used at their full potency. Examples of carrier oils that you can use are avocado oil, sweet almond oil or the very easily accessible olive oil. Each type of oil has different properties that make them a better match for certain skin and body conditions. Avocado oil is great for sensitive skin. Coconut oil will work wonders on hair that is dry or damaged. Oils with added vitamin E are often recommended because it acts as a natural preservative. Carrier oils have a tendency to become rancid with time and this will help prevent your product from expiring.

Another item that you will need to have to create the recipes are herbs. Some of the most common used herbs are spearmint, rosemary, basil and lavender. They possess fabulous healing properties. These can easily be purchased at your local grocery store or if you enjoy gardening, they can be grown right in your own backyard. It doesn't get much more organic than that! But just as oils are sometimes irritating to the skin, herbs can be as well. To do a spot test, simply rub the fresh herb on a small part of your arm. If the herb is dried, you will need to soak it in a little water first. If you don't notice any redness or irritation after twenty-four hours, the herb is safe for you to use.

You may also need some other common kitchen ingredients such as honey, avocado or baking soda. Most ingredients you can find at your local grocery store. Some may need to be purchased at a natural health specialty store and some may be only available online. You will also need some basic kitchen utensils. Measuring cups and spoons, mixing bowls and storage containers should be readily available. You will need an electric mixer, either a stand-up or handheld will work. You will also need a double boiler for several recipes. If you do not have one, simply make your own by placing a saucepan over a bowl of water to melt the necessary ingredients.

Most essential oils do not store well in plastic containers, so invest in dark tinted glass bottles. Most products that you will be making should also be stored in a dark and cool place to prevent bacteria from growing. Make sure that the containers and your hands are completely dry before storing your products.

Always sterilize any containers being used. If a product ends up having an odd smell after storage, it is recommended to dispose of the product as it may be bacteria infested. If the product is made with an ingredient that can spoil, it will need to be stored in the refrigerator and used by the time the ingredient would typically spoil.

By making your own bath and body products at home, you will experience radiant skin, free of irritation and redness. Since these products are antiseptic, you will have clearer skin with less breakouts. You will have the power of knowing what you are exposing your body to and you may even be able to save quite a bit of money. So, if you are ready to explore the world of homemade organic body care recipes, good luck!

I hope by now you've had a chance to make a few of the body care recipes. If you did then I think you will understand why I am so obsessed with making my own beauty care products. Not only do they feel and smell deliciously amazing, but they are so healthy you may just want to eat them.

Don't let the recipes overwhelm you. Just start out making your favorite body care products and your favorite scents to get started. Before you know it, you will be a pro at making your own beauty care products from home. You may even decide down the road to market them, who knows?

Whatever you do, don't be afraid to experiment with new combinations of oils and scents. It keeps things funs, exciting and unique. And don't be shy about sharing these recipes as gifts for birthdays and Christmas. Any time you are able to help someone make the move from the toxic, commercial beauty products that are tested on animals to healthy natural products that are aligned with nature- you are giving one of the greatest gifts you can give!

Lightning Source UK Ltd.
Milton Keynes UK
UKHW050626080123
414987UK00016B/301